CO-CREATIVE SCIENCE

CO-CREATIVE SCIENCE

*A REVOLUTION IN SCIENCE
PROVIDING REAL SOLUTIONS
FOR TODAY'S HEALTH &
ENVIRONMENT*

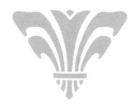

MACHAELLE SMALL WRIGHT

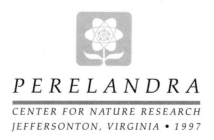

PERELANDRA

CENTER FOR NATURE RESEARCH
JEFFERSONTON, VIRGINIA • 1997

Manufactured in the United States of America

Designed by Machaelle Wright and James F. Brisson

Cover design by James F. Brisson

Copyedited by Elizabeth McHale

Desktop publishing layout by Machaelle Wright and Amy Shelton

This book was formatted, laid out and produced
using Corel Ventura 7 software along with
the Hewlett Packard Laser Jet 4 printer.

Printed on recycled paper

Published by Perelandra, Ltd.

P.O. Box 3603, Warrenton, VA 20188

Library of Congress Card Catalog Number: 97-067646

Wright, Machaelle Small

CO-CREATIVE SCIENCE:

A Revolution in Science

Providing Real Solutions for

Today's Health & Environment

ISBN: 0-927978-25-3

2 4 6 8 9 7 5 3 1

To Nature:
The best partner in science
and life that a person can have

Contents

Introduction

CONGRATULATIONS! UNLESS YOU already love science, you had to get over the dulling thud you experienced in your head when you read the word "science" on the front cover in order to open the book to this page. I guarantee that you won't be sorry. This actually *is* a book about science—a new science called "co-creative science." There are a number of things that make this science different from the "normal" science in our society that is called "contemporary science." You will learn about many of those differences as you read this book. But one of the exciting aspects of the new science is that everyone actively participates in it. It is not a spectator sport for everyone but the researchers. This is a science that you must personally apply to your life in order to experience its benefits. And it has *extraordinary* benefits for your health and for your environment. This is a science that you can use personally and it will make a difference—in your life and in the larger world.

Co-Creative Science is for scientists who are interested in exploring a new way to address the many serious problems that are mushrooming all around us, but it is also for the non-scientists who want to take charge of their lives in a positive, efficient and incredibly effective way.

The first and second chapters are written for both the scientists and non-scientists. They set the foundation for what co-creative science is and what makes it different. Chapters 3 and 4 are written for the scientists and science students. But I urge the non-scientists to read these two chapters, as well. They contain an explanation of the differences between contemporary and co-creative science, the differences in how the respective sciences function, and the training and credentials that are required for becoming a full-functioning co-creative scientist. Obviously, this information will be of special interest to scientists. But, it is important for non-scientists to learn about the education that is required of co-creative scientists. First of all, non-scientists have a role to play in co-creative science, and the more they learn about their scientists the better they will understand the role of both the scientists and non-scientists. Also, it is important that non-scientists know how to discern a qualified co-creative scientist from a co-creative scientist "imitator," one who talks a good game but doesn't actually know what he is doing. These imitators can lead non-scientists down a frustrating, time-consuming and disappointing path. Chapters 3 and 4 give non-scientists the needed yardstick for discerning well.

Chapter 5 is written especially for non-scientists. It describes the key role the non-scientist plays in co-creative science and how non-scientists can incorporate this co-creative science successfully into their lives. But I urge the scientists to read this chapter as well, because it is important for them to understand the role of non-scientists in the new science and how they (the scientists) can help the non-scientists fulfill that role, which, in turn, will be vital for the success of the co-creative scientist's work.

Co-Creative Science is also a book about nature. What makes this science unique is that it establishes a direct, active and personal partnership between you and nature for working together to successfully address the many problems—critical and not so critical—that pummel our everyday lives. Once you have finished reading this book, you will be convinced that, yes, there is an intelligence in nature, that this intelligence can be accessed by anyone who wishes and that together with this intelligence we can forge a partnership that can make *real* changes.

———————◆◆◆———————

Perelandra is a nature research center, founded in 1977, by Machaelle Small Wright. Her research is centered around learning about nature in new ways from nature itself. She works with nature intelligence in a conscious, coordinated and educational effort that has resulted in understanding and demonstrating a new approach to health, agriculture and environmental balance. This new approach involves creating a working partnership with nature that emphasizes balance and teamwork. The balance is a result of concentrating on the laws of nature and form. The teamwork is established between the individual and the levels of intelligence inherent in all of nature.

Machaelle Wright's laboratory and the primary focus of her work is the Perelandra garden where she works with nature to create an environment based on the principles of balance. In this laboratory, she and nature work together to apply the laws of nature in new ways that better address today's environmental and health issues.

As a result of the research with nature at Perelandra, a new science has been developed called "co-creative science." Traditional science is man's study of reality and how it works. Co-creative science is the study of reality and how it works from nature's perspective and by human and nature working together in a peer, balanced partnership.

CO-CREATIVE SCIENCE

When Magellan's expedition first landed at Tierra del Fuego, the Fuegans, who for centuries had been isolated with their canoe culture, were unable to see the ships anchored in the bay. The big ships were so far beyond their experience that, despite their bulk, the horizon continued unbroken: The ships were invisible. This was learned on later expeditions to the area when the Fuegans described how, according to one account, the shaman had first brought to the villagers' attention that the strangers had arrived in something which although preposterous beyond belief, could actually be seen if one looked carefully. We ask how they could not see the ships . . . they were so obvious, so real . . . yet others would ask how we cannot see things just as obvious.*

—JOHN W. MATTINGLY

---

* Mattingly, J. W. Foreword. In B. Lynes, *The Cancer Cure that Worked. Fifty Years of Suppression.* Marcus Books. Mexico. 1987.

1
Changing How We Perceive Nature

I N ORDER TO UNDERSTAND co-creative science and what
makes it unique, we need to understand nature in a deeper
and more comprehensive way. This is because what makes
co-creative science different from all other science is that it
involves working with nature in a conscious and direct manner. Let me explain. In contemporary science (the term used
for the science that is practiced today and with which we are
all familiar), the scientist attempts to discover how nature
works through testing and observation. He then draws conclusions about how nature works based on what he has observed
and understood. In co-creative science, the scientist acknowledges that there is an inherent intelligence within all of nature, builds a communication bridge that allows him to access
that intelligence, and then asks nature directly to explain and
provide experiential insight to him so that he may understand
"from the horse's mouth" (so to speak) how something works.
In co-creative science, nature becomes a fully operational,

functioning, conscious partner with the scientist. Together they create a team, with each member of the team providing specific and different information that is needed for understanding and solving a defined problem.

But to really understand co-creative science, we must first change how we perceive nature. The key to changing our understanding has to do with how we define nature itself. Usually, when we think of nature, we think of rocks, rivers, mountains, clouds, birds, trees, flowers. . . . But, after having worked as a co-creative scientist for over twenty years, I have learned that nature is actually much more than this.

In 1990, it was brought to my attention that when nature and I used the word "nature," we probably didn't assume the same definition. So, like a good co-creative scientist, I asked nature to define itself. (I describe how I bridge communication with nature in Chapter 4. For now, just pretend the words "I asked nature to define itself" are the most normal thing a person can say, and read on.) In order to understand their definition, nature said I had to first allow it to define form. I was surprised by the definition of both words.

FORM: *We consider reality to be in the form state when there is order, organization and life vitality* [initiates action] *combined with a state of consciousness. . . . We do not consider form to be only that which can be perceived by the five senses. In fact, we see form from this perspective to be extremely limited, both in its life reality and in its ability to function. We see form from the perspective of the five senses to be useful only for the most basic and fundamental level of identification. From this perspective, there is very little relationship to the full understanding and knowledge of how a unit or form system functions.*

All energy contains order, organization and life vitality; therefore, all energy is form. If one were to use the term "form" to identify that which can be perceived by the five senses and the word "energy" to refer to that aspect of an animal, human, plant or object's reality that cannot be readily perceived by the five senses, then one would be accurate in the use of these two words. However, if one were to use the word "form" to refer to that which can be perceived by the five senses and assume that form to be a complete unit of reality unto itself, and use the word "energy" to refer to a level beyond form, one would then be using these words inaccurately. From our perspective, form and energy create one unit of reality and are differentiated from one another solely by the individual's ability to perceive them with his or her sensory system. In short, the differentiation between form and energy within any given object, plant, animal or human lies with the observer.

On the planet Earth, the personality, character, emotional makeup, intellectual capacity, strong points and gifts of a human are all form. They are that which gives order, organization and life vitality to consciousness.

Order and organization are the physical structures that create a framework for form. In short, they define the walls. But we have included the dynamic of life vitality when we refer to form because one of the elements of form is action, and it is life vitality that initiates and creates action.

NATURE: *In the larger universe and beyond, on its many levels and dimensions, there are a number of groups of consciousness that, although equal in importance, are quite different in expression and function. Together, they make up the full expression of the larger, total life picture. No one piece, no one expression, can be missing or the larger life picture on all its levels and dimensions will cease to exist. One such consciousness has been universally termed "nature." Because of what we are saying about the larger picture not existing without all of its parts, you may assume that nature exists as both a reality and a consciousness on all dimensions and all levels. It cannot be excluded.*

*Each group of consciousness has an area of expertise. As we said, all groups are equal in importance but express and function differently from one another. These different expressions and functions are vital to the overall balance of reality. A truly symbiotic relationship exists among the groups and is based on balance—that is, universal balance. The human soul-oriented dynamic is **evolution** in scope and function. Nature is a massive, intelligent consciousness group that expresses and functions within the many areas of **involution**, that is, moving soul-oriented consciousness into any direction or level of form.*

*Nature is the conscious reality that supplies order, organization and life vitality for this shift. Nature is the consciousness that is, for your working understanding, intimately linked with form. Nature is the consciousness that comprises all form on all levels and dimensions. It **is** form's order, organization and life vitality. Nature is first and foremost a consciousness of equal importance with all other groups of* *consciousness in the largest scheme of reality. It expresses and functions uniquely in that it comprises all form on all levels and dimensions and is responsible for and creates all of form's order, organization and life vitality.*

Take a minute to think about this. Nature is saying that it is the order, organization and life vitality of all form and that all form contains consciousness. The first important point nature is making is that all form—that is, anything that has order, organization and life vitality—is nature. This goes way beyond the common notion that nature is trees, birds and rivers. This book is form. Its pages and ink are form. They have order, organization and the molecules contain life vitality. Therefore, this book, its pages and ink are all part of that consciousness and intelligence that is nature because nature supplies all order, organization and life vitality. The chair you are currently sitting in (assuming you are sitting) is nature. The walls surrounding you are nature. The windows that look out to the sky, birds and landscape are also nature. Everything in the room you are sitting in is nature.

As if this weren't enough, I'd like to expand this point by calling your attention to the Periodic Table of the Elements. (See table on the next page.) Look at it carefully. Every element listed in this chart is found within nature. They are the fundamental materials of which all matter is composed. Every element on this chart—every molecule—has its own order, organization and life vitality. By combining them, we get vinyl, Naugahyde, nylon, polyester—and even plastic. The materials for these products are all found in nature and are listed on the Periodic Table. It's just that they are combined

Periodic Table of Elements

period \ group	Ia	IIa	IIIb	IVb	Vb	VIb	VIIb		VIII		Ib	IIb	IIa	IVa	Va	VIa	VIIa	0
1	1 H hydrogen																1 H hydrogen	2 He helium
2	3 Li lithium	4 Be beryllium											5 B boron	6 C carbon	7 N nitrogen	8 O oxygen	9 F fluorine	10 Ne neon
3	11 Na sodium	12 Mg magnesium											13 Al aluminum	14 Si silicon	15 P phosphorus	16 S sulfur	17 Cl chlorine	18 Ar argon
4	19 K potassium	20 Ca calcium	21 Sc scandium	22 Ti titanium	23 V vanadium	24 Cr chromium	25 Mn manganese	26 Fe iron	27 Co cobalt	28 Ni nickel	29 Cu copper	30 Zn zinc	31 Ga gallium	32 Ge germanium	33 As arsenic	34 Se selenium	35 Br bromine	36 Kr krypton
5	37 Rb rubidium	38 Sr strontium	39 Y yttrium	40 Zr zirconium	41 Nb niobium	42 Mo molybdenum	43 Tc technetium	44 Ru ruthenium	45 Rh rhodium	46 Pd palladium	47 Ag silver	48 Cd cadmium	49 In indium	50 Sn tin	51 Sb antimony	52 Te tellurium	53 I iodine	54 Xe xenon
6	55 Cs cesium	56 Ba barium	57 La * lanthanum	72 Hf hafnium	73 Ta tantalum	74 W tungsten	75 Re rhenium	76 Os osmium	77 Ir iridium	78 Pt platinum	79 Au gold	80 Hg mercury	81 Tl thallium	82 Pb lead	83 Bi bismuth	84 Po polonium	85 At astatine	86 Rn radon
7	87 Fr francium	88 Ra radium	89 Ac ** actinium	104 Rf rutherfordium	105 Ha hahnium													

* 6

58 Ce cerium	59 Pr praseodymium	60 Nd neodymium	61 Pm promethium	62 Sm samarium	63 Eu europium	64 Gd gadolinium	65 Tb terbium	66 Dy dysprosium	67 Ho holmium	68 Er erbium	69 Tm thulium	70 Yb ytterbium	71 Lu letelium

** 7

90 Th thorium	91 Pa protactinium	92 U uranium	93 Np neptunium	94 Pu plutonium	95 Am americium	96 Cm curium	97 Bk berkelium	98 Cf californium	99 Es einsteinium	100 Fm fermium	101 Md mendelevium	102 No nobelium	103 Lr lawrencium

in a way that produces what we call vinyl, nylon, polyester and plastic.

For example: We would all probably agree that Dacron is not a natural fiber. It is a synthetic polyester fiber, and we don't harvest polyester fibers from the field. The following is the chemical makeup of Dacron:

$$\underrightarrow{\text{heat}} (OCH_2CH_2 - O - CO - \boxed{O} - CO -)Y + (Y - 1)H_2O$$
$$(C_6H_6)$$

y = 80 – 130
Molecular weight: 15,000 to 24,000

Dacron is nothing more than carbon (C), hydrogen (H) and oxygen (O), all elements found in nature, that have been specially combined in a lab by a process called polymerization. (Polymerization is a scientific term for the chemical process used to make grossly fat molecules.)

Some more examples:

Acetylene is an unsaturated hydrocarbon ($HC \equiv CH$). It is made up of hydrogen (H) and carbon (C). When you add to it chlorine (Cl), you get neoprene rubber. When you add nitrogen (N) to acetylene, you get an interestingly odd combination of products: fertilizers, weed killers and melamine plastics.

Ethylene ($H_2C = CH_2$) is also made up of hydrogen and carbon. Add acetylene to it and you produce acrylic fibers. Add both acetylene and chlorine to ethylene and you produce vinyl plastics.

Propylene is $H_3C - CH = CH_2$. From it we get plastics.

7

From butadiene ($H_2C = CH - CH = CH_2$) we get nitrite rubber and ABS plastics.

All of this is to show you that the matter that is combined in different ways to create synthetic materials can be found on the Periodic Table of the Elements, and everything listed on this chart may be found within nature.

Generally, when I bring up Dacron and plastic, a debate breaks out. Just because the elements exist and can be combined in this way, *should* we combine them? Isn't this manipulation of nature at its worst? And look at the mess these kinds of products have caused our ecology. I absolutely agree that just because we humans *can* figure out how to combine certain natural materials to create a new compound does not automatically mean the materials *should* be combined. All we have to do is look at the contents of a landfill to figure this out. But consider this: What if the chemist in his laboratory was working as a co-creative scientist in a conscious partnership with nature. The products that would come out of this lab would all be environmentally sound because nature would not consider a development that was out of balance with its immediate environment and the larger planetary environment. To operate in such an imbalanced manner would be contrary to everything that nature is and how it functions. So the chemist functioning as a co-creative scientist would be directed by nature to develop products that would address the issue at hand *and* be environmentally responsive. This is what co-creative science is all about.

The difficulty begins with how we perceive what constitutes nature: consider what we think when we use the terms "natural" and "unnatural." Generally, we consider something to be natural if it is a material or element that is found growing or existing on the planet that is then modified and used by humans. For example, raw cotton is harvested from the field, made into fiber threads that then become cloth. This eventually becomes a shirt. We consider an all-cotton shirt natural —yet you can't go out into a field and harvest a shirt. We consider something to be unnatural when two or more natural elements, such as carbon and hydrogen, are combined by man to create a compound that bears little or no resemblance to its original elements, such as vinyl. Other examples are cement, rayon, acrylic fiber and . . .

A garden. A garden is not natural. It is man-made. You don't go out in the wild and run across a free-growing vegetable garden containing cabbage, beans, tomatoes, snap peas and watermelon. We invented gardens. We got tired of all that hunting and foraging and decided to centralize our food supply. So we collected seed from various plants growing in the wild and planted the seed in one, easy-to-access location. Thus, we created something that did not previously exist.

I once read that someone said a garden is man's attempt to conquer nature. Whoever said this had a point. Generally, plants in the wild automatically grow where conditions are conducive to their growth. When they are centralized in a garden location, they are removed from their supportive environment and placed in an "unnatural" environment. This creates massive imbalance. Traditional and organic gardeners attempt to "conquer" the situation by restoring a balance that accommodates their definition of a garden and how it is to function. Co-creative gardeners work in a conscious partnership with nature, much as the co-creative scientist works with nature, to create an environmentally balanced biosphere on all levels —seen and unseen—that provides a new support system for all the plants and other life in that garden.

To sum up this first point about nature being all form: What I have grown to understand over the years is that when we speak of nature, we are talking about everything around us. The world of nature is not just relegated to parks, farms, countryside, animals and wilderness. It includes apartment buildings, asphalt, shopping malls and street corners.

The second important point nature is making in its definitions of form and nature is that in order for anything to be form, it must have consciousness combined with its order, organization and life vitality. This means that if you are holding some object in your hand and it has order, organization and life vitality, *it must also have consciousness*—otherwise, it would be beyond form and you would not be able to perceive it under any circumstances. And if it has consciousness, it has intelligence. If it has intelligence, it can communicate. If we can discover the common bridge between us for communication, we cannot only communicate our ideas and thoughts to this thing in our hand, but it can also communicate its information back to us. And it has something to communicate. It knows what it is, what defines its balance, what it needs to restore and maintain that balance at any given point in time, how it fits and functions in its immediate environment and how it connects with the larger picture—both on this planet and beyond. It is because of the quality and depth of this information that the co-creative scientist seeks a working partnership with nature in every aspect of his research and development.

INVOLUTION/EVOLUTION BALANCE

All consciousness (human and nature) on our planet seeks to reflect and flow perfectly and fully through form. It is a natural dynamic contained within all life. This brings me to something I call "involution/evolution balance" or "i/e balance."

I/E Balance

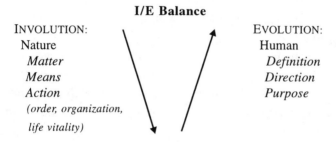

INVOLUTION:
Nature
Matter
Means
Action
(order, organization,
life vitality)

EVOLUTION:
Human
Definition
Direction
Purpose

Because nature supplies all form, and because all form has combined with it consciousness, all matter has inherent in it two dynamics: an *involution* dynamic (the matter, means and action) that is supplied by nature and an *evolution* dynamic (the definition, direction and purpose) that is supplied by consciousness. These two dynamics work in partnership, and, when left undisturbed, this partnership functions in balance. That is, the involution and evolution dynamics are synchronized with one another, thus creating a state of balance.

The following are examples of i/e balance.

In this first example, the evolution dynamic originates from the soul or devic level (a specific level of function within nature intelligence that is explained in Chapter 2) of an organism or object, and from this level the definition, direction and purpose are established. When considering trees, rocks, rivers, oceans and sky—objects that we would commonly consider "nature"—nature not only supplies the order, organization and life vitality (the involution dynamic) but also the consciousness or soul (the evolution dynamic). The i/e balance is contained within nature itself. The devic level of nature's intelligence supplies the consciousness or soul input and gives to a tree its definition, direction and purpose. The nature spirit level (another level of function within nature intelligence that is explained in Chapter 2) completes the i/e balance by supplying the matter, means and action for fulfilling the goals set by the definition, direction and purpose. The evolution dynamic in nature intelligence functions as the architect, drawing up the blueprints. The involution dynamic "builds" the structure according to the plans and maintains that structure throughout its full life cycle according to the patterns and rhythms set by nature's evolution dynamic. This is i/e balance as it is demonstrated in trees, mountains and clouds. What we see functioning before us is a full reflection of form's definition, direction and purpose.

A Tree's I/E Balance

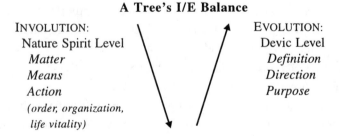

INVOLUTION:
Nature Spirit Level
Matter
Means
Action
(order, organization,
life vitality)

EVOLUTION:
Devic Level
Definition
Direction
Purpose

A Human Body's I/E Balance

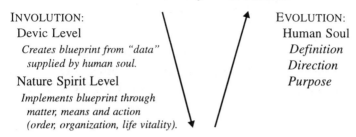

INVOLUTION:
  Devic Level
    Creates blueprint from "data"
    supplied by human soul.
  Nature Spirit Level
    Implements blueprint through
    matter, means and action
    (order, organization, life vitality).

EVOLUTION:
  Human Soul
    Definition
    Direction
    Purpose

The human body provides us with another example of i/e balance. The human soul establishes the definition, direction and purpose for a specific lifetime. Nature then provides the body according to that definition, direction and purpose. The devic level of nature intelligence creates the "blueprint" based on the soul information and the nature spirit level of nature intelligence implements these blueprints by providing the matter, means and range of action required by the soul. The result is that this soul has the physical vehicle to fully reflect and function according to its definition, direction and purpose. Throughout the person's full life cycle, the devic level modifies the makeup, patterns and rhythms according to however the person's soul modifies its original definition, direction and purpose. In other words, throughout a person's lifetime, there is a continuous communication between the human (evolution input) and the body's nature intelligence levels (involution input). A free-flowing communication between the two dynamics creates within us i/e balance and results in our having the body through which our soul may reflect and flow without constriction or interference. As a result, we experience what we call perfect health.

Nature's definition of "consciousness" and "soul" will help explain this interaction between the human soul and nature.

CONSCIOUSNESS: *The concept of consciousness has been vastly misunderstood. To put it simply, consciousness is the working state of the soul. In human expression, as one sees it demonstrated on the planet Earth, the personality, character, emotional makeup, intellectual capacity, strong points and gifts of a human are all form. They are that which give order, organization and life vitality to consciousness.*

We refer to the "working state of the soul" because there are levels of soul existence that are different than the working state and can best be described as a simple and complete state of being.

Humans tend to think of the soul as being something that exists far away from them because they are in form. This is an illusion. The core of any life is the soul. It cannot exist apart from itself. Like the heart in the human body, it is an essential part of the life unit. A human in form is, by definition, a soul fused with nature. Personality and character are a part of the nature/form package that allows the soul to function and to express itself in form. Personality and character are not the soul; they are the order and organization of that soul.

Human consciousness physically fuses into the body system first through the electrical system and then through the central nervous system and the brain. This is another aspect of nature supplying order, organization and life vitality. Consciousness itself cannot be measured or monitored as a reality. But what can be measured and monitored is the order, organization and life vitality of consciousness. Consciousness is the working state of the soul and is not form. It is nature, not consciousness, that supplies form.

We wish to add a thought here so that there will be no confusion about the relationship between nature and the human soul. Nature does not, with its own power, superimpose its interpretation of form onto a human soul. We have said that nature and the human soul are intimately and symbiotically related. This implies a give and take. No one consciousness group operates in isolation of the whole or of all other parts of the whole. When a soul chooses to move within the vast band of form, it communicates its intent and purpose to nature. It is from this that nature derives the specifics that will be needed for the soul to function in form. It is a perfect marriage of purpose with the order, organization and life vitality that is needed for the fulfillment of that purpose. Nature, therefore, does not define purpose and impose it on a human soul. It orders, organizes and gives life vitality to purpose for expression in form.

SOUL: *It is most difficult to define soul since—at its point of central essence—the soul is beyond form. Consequently, it is beyond words. However, it is not beyond any specific life form. As we have said, an individual is not separate or distant from his or her soul. Souls, as individuated life forces, were created and fused with form at the moment of the Big Bang.* Beyond form, souls are also beyond the notion of creation. So we refer to the moment of the Big Bang in terms*

---

* The Big Bang: The gigantic explosion in which the universe, as we know it, began. According to scientists, it occurred between 12 and 20 billion years ago. It brought about two major dynamics: individuation and the fusion of soul to form.

*of the soul, since this gives you a description of soul that will
be most meaningful to you. The Big Bang was the nature-
designed order, organization and life force used to differenti-
ate soul into sparks of individuated light energy. . . .*

The glitch to our human i/e balance is free will. We can
make our free will jump right into the middle of i/e balance
and use it to distort our intuitive understanding of the soul's
definition, direction and purpose. What if we got a glimpse of
this soul information and, for whatever reason, decided we
didn't like it. We wanted a different life. Suppose we perceive
that the life based on the information as we understood it
would be too tough or too tedious. So we insert our will right
into the middle of the i/e balance and we modify that evolution information according to our preference and desire. Now
nature has two sets of definitions, directions and purposes to
deal with. The operating devic blueprint will still reflect the
soul's original definition, direction and purpose. However, we
are now consciously operating with another set of definition,
direction and purpose—the free will set. As we move through
our daily lives, we override the soul information with our
conscious desires and we find that things are not moving too
smoothly through this body. This is because we are trying to
move one set of evolutionary dynamics through a body that
was designed for another set—the soul set. We are no longer
operating within i/e balance and we will experience all kinds
of health issues as a result.

Because of free will, i/e balance is a difficult dynamic for
us to maintain. We frequently jump into the middle of it. For
us, i/e balance rests not only on our ability to trust in the

movement of our own soul, but also in our ability to consciously translate and perceive our soul's definition, direction
and purpose and not use our free will to try to manipulate our
soul. This is one of the things we are here on Earth to learn:
the marrying of our conscious selves to our souls and the full
fusion of this with our physical bodies. I am not implying that
consciously achieving our i/e balance is easy. I'm only using
an example that is familiar to us all in order to make i/e balance more easily understood. Well, actually, if it was just left
up to our soul and nature, we would experience perfect i/e
balance easily. It's free will that adds the elements of excitement, confusion and challenge. As we develop and discipline
our free will, we expand our understanding to include the
wisdom to know when and how to appropriately apply free
will, and our experience of i/e balance will be unencumbered
and beyond words.

Another example of i/e balance is the balance that is at the
heart of our co-creative partnership with nature. There are
many different kinds of gardens: herb gardens, rock gardens,
perennial gardens, wildflower gardens, Japanese moss gardens, Zen sand gardens . . . and vegetable gardens. When you
are working directly in partnership with nature, you cannot
simply announce, "Let's put in a garden!" and expect that
you will get any information back from nature regarding the
garden. You must supply the definition, direction and purpose
of this garden. In other words, you must supply the evolution
dynamic within the i/e balance, and you are the only one who
can do that. Nature will not do your job for you. It will only
supply the evolution dynamic for objects that fall within its

A Garden's I/E Balance

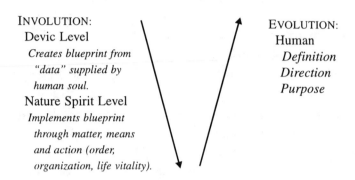

INVOLUTION:
Devic Level
Creates blueprint from
"data" supplied by
human soul.
Nature Spirit Level
Implements blueprint
through matter, means
and action (order,
organization, life vitality).

EVOLUTION:
Human
Definition
Direction
Purpose

"natural" domain: plants, rocks, deer, lightning, etc. It does not supply the evolution dynamic for form that falls outside this natural domain, such as gardens. Remember, gardens are a man-made invention. In a co-creative partnership with nature, when you decide you want to create a garden, you are responsible for supplying the evolution dynamic: definition, direction and purpose.

Nature creates the blueprints according to your evolution input, and it is only after this information is supplied by you that the devic level of nature intelligence can establish the blueprint for your garden. Based on your definition (a vegetable garden), direction (a vegetable garden in my backyard that includes succession planting so that we may harvest from it year round), and purpose (a garden that feeds daily my family of six—my two teenage sons, my ten-year-old daughter, my two-year-old son, my wife and myself), nature creates the order, organization and life vitality patterns and rhythms that will best respond to the information you have supplied.

Why would you go through all of this trouble? Why would you want to establish a co-creative partnership in the first place? Well, once you have supplied a good definition, direction and purpose for your garden, nature will design and implement with you a garden that will be *in balance*. And this is why you go through all that trouble. When you have balance, as in the human body, everything operates smoothly and is synchronized. No more guesswork. No more trying one trick after another in order to achieve success. And the quality of food that comes from such a garden contains the same balance that is reflected in the garden.

Once we establish a co-creative partnership with nature, we have the finest experts in what needs to occur in order to achieve and maintain balance. One of the most difficult things a person new to a co-creative partnership has to learn is not to try to do nature's job. We are very used to deciding what we wish to accomplish (evolution) and then *also* deciding the best way to achieve our goals and the best materials to use (involution). But *equal partnership* does not mean that we are equally capable of doing nature's job. It means our role in the partnership is equal to nature's role—but the two roles are very different. In a balanced partnership, these two roles function together *equally*. The first trick to working with nature to achieve i/e balance is to do our job well and then let nature supply the matter, means and action for accomplishing the defined goal. At first blush, it seems like a co-creative partnership is more work than it's worth. In actuality, it takes a tremendous burden off our shoulders. Many people who have entered such a partnership have talked to me about the weight that has been lifted from them. They no longer have to think of everything themselves. For example, gardeners now have a partner who can tell them the best location for their garden, what vegetables to plant, where to plant them, what interplanting to do, when to plant, when to thin, when to water and how much. . . . And all of that information has balance. This spells success.

Sometimes people assume that a co-creative relationship with nature means that they announce the definition, direction and purpose of their garden and then sit back, beer in hand, and watch nature spirits run around doing all the work. After all, I am saying that nature supplies the matter, means and action. Doesn't this mean that in a garden nature manifests the right tools and then gets out there and starts turning soil? *No.* It's a *working partnership.* Nature gives us the information that is needed to create this garden in balance. That includes what tools are best for achieving our goal in light of the variables, working conditions and our ability. For example, nature won't suggest that your four-year-old help dig a sandbox area with a front-end loader. It will suggest the kind of tool that will be safe for this child to use that will also allow him a successful experience as he helps you with the digging. Nature gives you this information because it takes all the variables into account in light of your stated goal and establishes the *balanced* way to proceed. In short, nature doesn't do the work for you. It works *with* you.

I have said that there are many kinds of gardens. Many do not grow in soil. In 1993, I asked nature to define a garden.

From nature's perspective, a garden is any environment that is initiated by humans, given its purpose, definition and direction by humans, and maintained with the help of humans. For nature to consider something to be a garden, we must see humans actively involved in all three of these areas. It is the human who calls for a garden to exist. Once the call is made, nature responds accordingly to support that defined call because a garden exists through the use of form.

Humans tend to look at gardens as an expression of nature. Nature looks at gardens as an expression of humans. They are initiated, defined and maintained by humans. When humans dominate all aspects and elements of the life of the garden, we consider this environment to be human dominant. We consider an environment to be "nature friendly" when humans understand that the elements used to create gardens are form and operate best under the laws of nature, and when humans have the best intentions of trying to cooperate with what they understand these laws to be. When humans understand that nature is a full partner in the design and operation of that environment—and act on this knowledge—we consider the environment to be actively moving toward a balance between involution (nature) and evolution (human).

As a result, the nature-friendly environment supports and adds to the overall health and balance of all it comprises as well as the larger whole. It also functions within the prevailing laws of nature (the laws of form) that govern all form on the planet and in its universe. In short, when a garden operates in a balance between involution and evolution, it is in step with the overall operating dynamics of the whole; the various parts that comprise a garden operate optimally, and the garden as a whole operates optimally.

Nature does not consider the cultivation of a plot of land as the criteria for a garden. Nature considers a garden to exist wherever humans define, initiate and interact with form to create a specialized environment. This is the underlying intent of a garden and the reason behind the development of specialized environments such as vegetable gardens. Nature applies the word "garden" to any environment that meets these criteria. It does not have to be growing in soil. It only needs to be an environment that is defined, initiated and appropriately maintained by humans.

This is what nature means when it uses the word "garden." The laws and principles that nature applies in the co-creative vegetable garden are equally applicable to any kind of garden, whether it is growing in soil or otherwise. . . . The principles and processes apply across the board because all gardens are operating with the same dynamics—only the specific form elements that make up each garden have changed.

What are some of these other specialized environments or soil-less gardens? According to nature, a garden has just three criteria: It is initiated by humans, given its definition, direction and purpose by humans, and maintained with the help of humans. Well, managed forests, landscaping, farms, and potted plants would also be gardens that grow in soil. Soil-less gardens could include waterways, ponds, the atmosphere, aquariums, livestock ranches, trout farms, a landscaping business, a swimming pool, a home, large and small businesses,

individual offices within a business, a classroom, a depart-
ment, a college study program, a children's playground, an
assembly line, a car, a computer, a computer program, a
human body, a printing company, the space shuttle, a toxic
waste dump, a nuclear waste storage facility, community
landfills, parking lots, national parks, the New Jersey Turn-
pike, an AIDS research lab, a pharmaceutical research and development lab, a police crime lab, athletic training programs,
a movie production company, an artist's work. . . . All of
these soil-less "environments" meet the criteria for a garden.
This is actually good news. In order to establish a co-creative
partnership with nature, you won't have to give up your present life, quit your job and buy land in the country. Stay right
where you are. Remember, where there is form, there is nature. Where nature and humans interact, there is a garden.
Where there is a garden, there is an implied co-creative partnership. And where there is a co-creative partnership, there is
the potential for i/e balance.

2

What Is Nature Intelligence?

ANOTHER GOOD TITLE FOR this chapter could be "Meet Your Partner" because the partnership in co-creative science is between a human and nature intelligence. When an individual creates this partnership, he is not creating it with a tree or a rock or a bird. He is developing the partnership with the intelligence that is inherent in that tree, rock or bird.

One of the first problems we face when we attempt to establish a co-creative connection with nature is the assumption that nature intelligence operates and has the same properties as our own intelligence. Generally, this happens because the only intelligence we are familiar with is human intelligence and we have been made to believe that the only existing intelligence is human intelligence. Over the many years I have been working with nature intelligence, I have learned well that it is different from my own. By different, I certainly don't mean to imply that it is threatening or powerful in ways that could be harmful to me. To the contrary, I have always felt completely at ease, safe and comfortable with this intelligence. It's just that it's unlike anything I have previously experienced. It *is* powerful, but the only way I can accurately describe this to you is to say that it feels like *balanced power*. When I am connected with this intelligence, I can feel that it is constantly taking into account my present state of mind and being. I can literally feel nature's intelligence dynamic shift and adjust to me. As a result, I never feel overwhelmed by it.

In 1996, I decided it was time to address the issue of nature intelligence with nature directly. It was a bit like turning to my long-time partner and saying, "Explain yourself." The following is what nature said.

In general, intelligence as a dynamic is above and beyond human traits defined by the sensory system and the human ability to communicate with others. It is a part of all life, and one may say that it is the organizing dynamic between the form of that life and its soul. Note the word "organizing." Because nature is the order, organization and life vitality of all form, it is accurate to say that nature plays a key role in the intelligence in all life—all form. Intelligence as a dynamic is much broader than what has been defined by humans. Their definition is but a drop in the bucket, as you say.

Intelligence is beyond the human brain. Consequently, it does not require form to provide a specific physical facility, such as the human brain, for it to be present and to function. It only requires that there be a focal point (the form itself) through which intelligence may flow. It does not need a central nervous system, a sensory system or a brain. Again, it needs only the overall form focal point in order to flow. We

*have used the word "flow" twice now, and this is a key to un-
derstanding intelligence as a dynamic. It is an organizing
flow from the soul to a physical focal point, and it flows
through the form. It does not require that it be held, sorted,
identified and catalogued. It simply flows.*

*What all form has in common is its intelligence. This dy-
namic is common in makeup and flow. How it expresses the
flow is determined by the unique qualities of the form itself.
All form must have intelligence in order to exist because all
form must be linked with and express its soul dynamics. Intelligence is the organizing dynamic that provides the movement
of soul through form. Intent and intuition[1]* [see notes at the end
of this chapter] *are but two of the qualities within this massive,
driving dynamic called intelligence. If you could see and feel
this dynamic, you would experience an active, driving force
moving throughout all creation that in size, scope and power
would be beyond words—and, from the perspective of the
Earth level, beyond belief. How* [many] *humans . . . express
and understand intelligence is limiting true intelligence to its
smallest point.*

MSW: Tell me more about the soul.

*At the time of the Big Bang,[2] the force of all reality indi-
viduated. When we use the word "individuated," people tend
to think that every single element of form came to exist as independent impulses. This is a misconception. The force of all
reality individuated into "packages," as it were, that contain
all the potential and all the elements needed for the full evolution that is required by the package itself. For humans, the
individuated soul[3] is made up of a package that contains all*

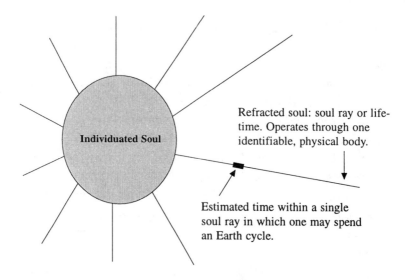

Refracted soul: soul ray or lifetime. Operates through one identifiable, physical body.

Individuated Soul

Estimated time within a single soul ray in which one may spend an Earth cycle.

the elements required for each refracted soul[3] in all its stages to move fully through evolution, and eventually return to and become part of the larger individuated soul again.

When one considers the countless range of different refracted lives through which the individuated soul operates, one may get an idea of how large each package is. If you wish to visualize the scope of human packages, imagine every element of nature, from its largest whale or mountain to its smallest proton. Then multiply this by one thousand. From this you will begin to get an idea of the scope of each human package. Once every refracted reflection that is part of the individuated soul has completed its evolution and "returned" to its larger soul reality (the individuated soul), it is conceivable that the individuated soul will then be prepared for its return to its pre–Big Bang existence.

One may say, then, that a form's soul is that massive dynamic that contains all potential and possibility. In short, it defines that form's full and complete evolution. A package contains all elements of the soul.

MSW: How does free will fit into this?

Free will applies to humans. Their (human) packages are fully involution/evolution (i/e) balanced. At the time of the Big Bang, the package was simultaneously fused with intelligence. In the case of humans, the Big Bang fused nature reality with human reality through the dynamic of intelligence. Because of free will, which is part of a human's package, a person has the ability at any time to consciously and willfully operate "outside" his own package. The potential for this is also part of the package. The human package supplies the full range and scope of free will impulses that include the ability to make conscious decisions to step beyond or outside one's own soul dynamic.

Because of free will, humans may deny the normal give-and-take between form (their person) and soul. As you might imagine, it is a serious situation when this occurs. But a major part of human evolution is conscious living. One cannot attain this state without free will, and one cannot have full free will without having the capability of denying (as well as accepting) any element of one's own being. However, free will goes beyond just denial of one's essential self. It includes stepping outside one's soul dynamic and embracing other elements in reality that are not compatible with oneself and one's soul. For there to be complete free will, there must be complete freedom.

Let us go on to nature intelligence. We have said that all form has its intelligence in common. By this we mean that the organizing dynamic between all form and its packages may be viewed as similar. This is critical for humans to understand because it is the reason they may interface and interact with the intelligence of anything around them. You may say that the intelligence of something operates within a universal framework, thus allowing for full and complete interchange. Nature intelligence is the organizing dynamic between the package of nature and its multitude of varying form. Consequently, when one connects with this flow, one accesses the full reality, potential and possibility of all of nature.

With each major classification of form there is a key element within its intelligence that defines it, making it unique with respect to every other classification. With human form, the key element is free will. With nature, the key element is inherent balance. Nature reality does not contain free will, and human reality does not contain inherent balance. The organization flow (the intelligence) of nature's soul dynamic moves through its many forms reflecting inherent balance—always.

When humans impact nature adversely, they do not disrupt nature reality on its intellectual level. They do, however, interfere with its reality on the form level. An out-of-balance condition within nature occurs when a balanced nature form has been altered by humans. Its intelligence level is still fused with that form and maintains inherent balance. Humans cannot impact this intelligence level. They may only access it.

When humans consider solutions for restoring balance to an out-of-balance world, they need only access the intelligence of the nature involved for answers. That intelligence *contains inherent balance and is fully capable of defining all that is required for reflecting that inherent balance through specific form.*

The biggest hurdle for humans in understanding nature intelligence is the habit of using human intelligence as the defining yardstick for the different intelligences in the rest of reality. Human intelligence is only one expression of intelligence. It is defined by the unique physical facility of human form through which human intelligence generally functions (brain, central nervous system and sensory system) and the overall driving dynamic of free will. Free will requires the development of intellectual characteristics such as the ability to think, consider, debate, argue, observe, develop opinions, educate and inform oneself, believe, daydream, fantasize, understand, define, discern, interpret and hypothesize. Within nature intelligence—where there is no free will but there is inherent balance—these characteristics are not needed. Nature intelligence operates in a state of being and constantly within present time. Because of inherent balance, nature intelligence does not need to develop the same characteristics as humans. Nature simply knows. It does not need the facilities for understanding what it knows and why.

In order for man to acknowledge and interface directly with nature intelligence, he must put aside the criteria that make up human intelligence and create bridges through which the two different intelligences may directly interface. Man must understand something about his own intelligence, how it operates, the range of its operation and what must be supplied in order to meet the needs of that range. He must then extend himself out to an intelligence with a different operation, range and need, and discover together with that intelligence a common meeting ground in which both may communicate. At Perelandra, examples of this are the use of kinesiology[4] as a communication tool between both intelligences (human and nature) and the various processes[5] that have been developed for mutually beneficial work to be done in partnership. Kinesiology and the numerous co-creative processes build a common framework through which the human and nature intelligences may work.

From the human perspective, accessing nature intelligence is a mystery. It does not respond to the kind of research that humans use in order to learn about and understand their own intelligence. For a human, nature intelligence is like a 5,000-piece puzzle that has been dumped in a great heap on the table before him. He has no idea what the picture is or how and where to begin to access it. Nature, of course, knows the picture and has its copy of the puzzle already put together. From nature's perspective, everything is in order. To work with nature intelligence, as we have said, man must learn to access it in an orderly fashion that meets the needs of his own intelligence. For example, he must devise mutually agreed upon "codes." A language must be developed that contains mutually agreed upon definitions.

Nature does not use or need words. At all times, nature knows. It does not need words to convey within nature what it knows. However, language becomes the bridge between the two intelligences. And it only succeeds when the differences between the intelligences are recognized and addressed. It fails when humans expect nature to understand and use language as you humans do.

One example of the language bridge is the widespread use by humans of the words "deva" and "nature spirit." "Deva" generally applies to that area of nature intelligence that operates in its architectural or creative mode. Because nature knows the intent and definition of this word when an individual uses it, its use allows that individual to access this area of nature's intelligence. The word is automatically matched with that area of nature intelligence that corresponds with its agreed upon definition. "Deva of Broccoli" connects the person with that area of nature intelligence that deals with the creative elements of the plant known as broccoli. Connecting with the Deva of Broccoli will not give you access to the creative level of intelligence that addresses kumquats. Nature responds in inherent balance. Therefore, connecting to the area dealing with kumquats when you request broccoli will not be nature's response.

"Nature spirit" generally applies to the action and implementation of the intelligence that functions unique to individual form within its (form's) context. The intelligence input about the fertilizing needs of broccoli growing in Kansas, Brazil and Israel will differ because the broccoli in each location is in a different context. The creative devic scope of nature intelligence is universal in its function. The nature spirit aspect focuses that intelligence on specific form within individual context and is, consequently, regional.

Because of the mutual understanding of the terminology by many people, humans may use these two terms to access areas of nature intelligence that operate within the definitions of the terms themselves. "Deva" and "nature spirit" allow an individual to link in an organized manner different pieces of *the puzzle that has been heaped on the table before them. However, if an individual chooses to switch these definitions—"nature spirit" would mean creativity and universality and "deva" would address implementation and action within context—accessing nature's intelligence would not be effective because there is no mutual agreement about changing the definitions.*

Someone may wish not to use these two terms at all. Perhaps he would prefer to use the word "plipcock" to refer to the creative areas of the intelligence and "mangoby" to refer to action and implementation in context. He cannot assume that nature intelligence automatically acknowledges and "records" these changes simply because he has thought of them and/or written down the new words and definitions. All this is an exercise of human intelligence. To create a language bridge using these two new words, he must directly address nature intelligence and "enter" the new terminology and definitions. He must then make sure nature accepts the new words.

Nature does not make judgments regarding specific words. It does not say, "Gee, we would have preferred 'mango' and 'persimmon.'" This kind of preference is demonstrated within human intelligence. Nature needs to know what humans mean when they use their own terms. If nature "rejects" the new words, it is not because of preference. It is because the definition is not clear enough for nature to know what you mean when you use these words. It requires you to be clearer than you have ever been. In short, words such as "deva" and "nature spirit" are used to access and address specific levels and areas in those levels within nature intelligence. They are mutually agreed upon access codes. When speaking about nature intelligence, these kinds of words do not refer to individual, independent beings within nature.

This brings us to the issue of elves, fairies, gnomes and devic angels. Nature intelligence does not include these types of beings. It is a massive intelligence, a dynamic. It is not made up of individual life forms. This intelligence dynamic flows through form. It is not made up of these forms. One may, however, look at beings such as elves and devic angels as communication bridges between man and nature intelligence. If nature is to communicate what it knows to an individual, it may create form through which this communication can flow. Nature is, after all, the order, organization and life vitality of all form. At any time, it may create, modify and utilize form in response to the moment. The "appearance" of a nature spirit is a response to the inherent balance of the moment that includes an individual human being. More often than not, the nature spirit form used is seen only within the mind's eye of the person with whom nature wishes to communicate. However, whether seen within the mind's eye or by the individual's outer sensory system, the form is equally real. But it is a communication bridge in the form of an elf, not an elf with an independent life of its own. The nature spirit level of nature's consciousness does not need elves and gnomes to function. That level simply flows through all existing form directly. When such an event occurs, many humans unfortunately tend to overlay it with expectation and definition that is unique to human intelligence rather than understand that this is a bridge from nature intelligence. It has different dynamics and has been initiated and activated for a specific purpose. If humans could focus on the communication surrounding such an event rather than get lost in the excitement of the event itself, more would come of the experience; and it would be more useful to them, as well.

The name "Pan" is used by humans to access and work with the part of nature intelligence that bridges the creative activity (devic) with the action and implementation activity (nature spirit) of the intelligence. The Pan function of nature intelligence also bridges these two activities with the overall soul dynamics of nature. Humans call these soul dynamics "natural law" or "laws of nature." The Pan function is critical because it operates as a switching station for the various levels of nature intelligence to "meet and mix." The Pan function organizes the flow in ways that are not found elsewhere in the larger nature intelligence. Because of its unique qualities within the overall dynamic flow, the Pan function may be accessed independently by humans and it may create a bridge on its own to communicate its unique knowledge to humans; hence, the experiences and sightings people have had with the forms they call "Pan."

It is through the Pan function that one finds the "heart of nature." This is because the Pan function mixes all levels of nature creativity with action and implementation, and then combines this mixture with its soul dynamics. In essence, by combining the soul dynamics, it provides the foundation for all nature intelligence—that is, inherent balance—as a result of its unique function. It is the action of bridging the combined levels with the soul dynamics that creates a different reality referred to as the "heart of nature."

When an individual connects with the Pan function within nature intelligence, he is linked with a most vibrant and comprehensive knowledge that is a result of this mixing and bridging activity. It is not the pure knowledge of the creative devic functions, nor is it the pure knowledge of the action and implementation functions. It is the knowledge that is created when these two functions combine to create a new, more complex reality; and then bridged to nature's soul dynamics, they create an even more complex reality.

Once the mixing and bridging of the various levels with one another and with the soul dynamics has occurred, the Pan function instantaneously shifts this new reality into its appropriate form. It is the Pan function that actually fuses nature intelligence with its form. Once fused, it is seated and stabilized. The intelligence-fused form is then maintained in its day-to-day rhythms primarily by the appropriate nature spirit level within the overall intelligence. To repeat: The appropriate devic and nature spirit functions for a specific form reality are combined by the Pan function. This combined reality is bridged to the soul dynamics. The intelligence that is fused into form is this complex mixture.

The Pan mixture does not reconnect with the pure nature spirit level of its intelligence until after the intelligence fuses with form. The fusion activates the nature spirit-level connections that are appropriate to this particular functioning form mixture. This ensures that only those elements that apply to a specific form are linked with and activated for that form. (This is the action of inherent balance.) Thus, you will not have elements within the nature spirit level of intelligence that are appropriate for snow linked with and activated for the *daily maintenance of a broccoli plant. This mixing/bridging/ release/fusion to the form and relinking process is one way nature intelligence organizes itself and functions in an appropriate and orderly fashion.*

When the Pan function is included in conings (as is the case with the conings that have been set up for the Perelandra processes and programs),[6] it introduces the dynamics of this vital activity within nature intelligence into the coning mix. Consequently, the coning dynamic includes the full mixing/bridging/release/fusion/relinking process. If an individual chooses to include only one "already identified" nature spirit element in a coning, he is eliminating the actual Pan function of the process. He has only a pre–Pan-function nature spirit link and/or a post–Pan-function link in the coning, depending on the definition of the name that is used for the specific nature spirit element. If he includes Pan, he automatically includes the appropriate nature spirit functions prior to the Pan function/operation and the nature spirit connection that occurs after the fusion of intelligence to form has taken place, plus the vital dynamic of the Pan function itself. Placing Pan into a coning automatically covers all the bases and makes for a stronger, more stable coning.

We would like to address the animal kingdom, for it is this area of nature where nature intelligence expresses itself most closely with human intelligence. Notice we said "expresses itself most closely" and did not say that the two intelligences were identical or related in any way. Within the animal kingdom, the underlying dynamic of intelligence is still inherent balance. Often this is demonstrated through instinct. Animals act on instinct. The fact that the animal kingdom includes brains, central nervous systems and sensory systems does not mean that it functions with free will. It does mean, however, that animals, because they have similar means of receiving and expressing stimuli, are more able to communicate what they know directly with humans in a way that is similar or familiar to humans. Oak trees simply do not have the same five senses for communicating with humans that a wolf or cat does. In short, oak trees don't have lips.

An animal may express what it knows at any given moment through its sensory system. It also receives information about what is presently going on in its environment through its sensory system. Consequently, an individual may understand what an animal knows through its eyes, its touch, its sounds. This does not mean an animal has intelligence traits identical to human traits simply because it can express what it knows through its eyes. Animals do not think, consider, debate, believe, daydream, understand, define or hypothesize. They don't need to. They know, and what they know is based on inherent balance and is expressed instinctually.

Animals that closely interface with humans (companion animals) also operate according to inherent balance. However, their environment and daily rhythms are defined by humans. Their instincts are expressed, but within the context of a human world. When there is a successful relationship between human and animal, the individual provides the environment and daily rhythm that takes into consideration and best suits the animal's ability to reflect inherent balance within the context of the individual's defined environment. In short, the two very different needs are expressed within one environment that is provided by man. (Conversely, in the wild, the animal provides the environment's operating "rules" for animals that the human adjusts to.) When the relationship between man and companion animal is not successful, man has provided an environment that is to his own liking but does not allow the animal to express its inherent balance. The animal's daily rhythms are defined and dictated solely by the individual, and the animal often expresses behavior that humans call "neurotic"—but the behavior is in response to the lack of balance.

It is important that man understand that the differences between human and nature intelligence remain the same when referring to animals. Animals are not creatures with one foot in the nature world and one foot in the human world. When an individual confuses this issue and looks at animals as furred or feathered humans, he misses the opportunity to interface with nature intelligence through form with a brain, central nervous system and sensory system that are similar to his own. This similarity between animals and humans enables humans to experience nature intelligence more easily. The similar physical makeup between man and animal doesn't mean the intelligences are similar. It only means that some of the ways of expressing the respective intelligences are similar.

People with companion animals may say that their animals have the ability to argue, observe, educate, decide and understand—all aspects of human intelligence. A fight to establish or maintain dominance does not meet the criteria of a human argument. The ability to see does not equal the ability to observe. Evolutionary development based on opportunities presented in an animal's environment and survival instincts does *not constitute education. Acting on instinct does not equal the ability to make decisions. And knowing that is based on inherent balance is not the same as understanding. With each intellectual trait individuals observe in animals that appears similar to human intellectual traits, they must view the animal trait from the perspective of inherent balance and the human trait from the perspective of free will. Only then will humans begin to understand the true differences between the traits and how they are expressed. And it is then that humans will begin to learn and understand something about the intelligence, which is so different from their own, that is called "nature intelligence."*

————————◆ ◆ ◆————————

NOTES

1. Intent: The conscious awareness of soul purpose, what is required within the scope of form to achieve soul purpose, and how the two function as a unit.

   Intuition: The communication bridge between the unconscious and the conscious. Intuition enables what is known on the level of the unconscious to be incorporated with and become a part of one's consciousness.

2. The Big Bang: The gigantic explosion in which the universe, as we know it, began. According to scientists, it occurred between 12 and 20 billion years ago. The Big Bang brought about two major dynamics: individuation and the fusion of soul to form.

3. Individuated soul: Individuated souls operate beyond time and space. Time and space are but two kinds of order and organization.

There can be form reality without time and space. Individuated souls are in a form reality that does not include time and space.

Refracted soul: In order to participate within many levels and dimensions, the individuated soul must modify itself to accommodate time and space. To do this, the soul creates what have been commonly called "lifetimes." At Perelandra, these are called "soul rays." The individuated soul refracts itself into a smaller unit that includes all of the qualities necessary for experiencing within a specific range of time and space. Each individuated soul has countless such refractions that are functioning in concert with it at all times.

4. Kinesiology is another name for muscle testing. For learning kinesiology and how to use it, see the appendix.

5. As a result of the co-creative research at Perelandra, a number of processes and programs have been developed that facilitate humans and nature working together to accomplish a common goal. Examples include the Energy Cleansing Process, the Battle Energy Release Process, the Calibration Process, MAP and the Microbial Balancing Program.

6. A coning is an i/e balanced vortex of conscious intelligent energy that has been activated by a human for a specific purpose when it is necessary for that individual to work with more than one intelligence simultaneously.

3

Co-Creative Science and the Co-Creative Scientist

SEVERAL YEARS AGO, I ASKED for the definition of science. Although the definition was several paragraphs long, it boiled down to one succinct sentence: *Science is the study of reality and how it works.* I then asked for the definition of co-creative science.

CO-CREATIVE SCIENCE: *The nature research at Perelandra is an example of co-creative science because it involves intelligence on two levels. On the one hand, we have reality as understood by the human soul; on the other hand, we have reality as understood by nature. This particular connection is especially vital because all life, as expressed in form, is the coming together of these two levels.*

For reality in form to function in balance and with a full and wide range of options, there must be not only the coming

*together of soul and matter, but there must also be under-
standing of the soul dynamic and how it works, and the nature dynamic and how that works. In addition, there must be
understanding of the combined soul/nature dynamic and how
it works as a unit. Up to the present time, the scientific community on the Earth level has separated the study of soul dynamics from nature dynamics. It has created two separate
schools: the evolutionary, human-dominant school in which
the human potential is studied; and the evolutionary, nature-
dominant school that studies the natural sciences.*

*To understand reality and how it works within form on the
Earth level, the two schools must be connected. But the necessary connection cannot be found in the two schools as they
are presently set up. That connection lies in the unit of the
soul dynamic and the nature dynamic as expressed in all
form. If one is to understand reality and how it works on the
Earth level, one must focus on reality as demonstrated in the
soul/form unit. The key to the next major scientific study is in
this focus. . . .*

In order for me to define co-creative science, I will describe some key elements of contemporary science and its scientists so that you may have something for comparison. But
first I'd like to make my personal position about contemporary science clear. I am not categorically opposed to contemporary science or its scientists. However, I question the
overall usefulness of contemporary science because it is not
balanced—that is, it does not include nature's input nor does
it maintain a faithfulness to the laws of nature. Therefore, it
cannot be fully responsive to today's needs, nor can it address

today's needs without setting into motion problems we will have to deal with in the future.

Contemporary and co-creative scientists have different attitudes and a different approach to science. These influence how the two groups think and function. How they think and function influences the quality of their work. My concern about contemporary scientists is not personal. Many are dedicated to trying to do something positive about the serious problems of the world. Despite their best intentions, the quality of their work unintentionally perpetuates the problems that face all of us today and cloud our future.

The following will help clarify the differences between contemporary science and its scientist and co-creative science and the co-creative scientist.

THE CONTEMPORARY SCIENTIST is acknowledged, by himself and others, as having reached a certain level of intellectual and practical training that defines what is legitimate and acceptable by his peers and enables him, through his research, to "figure out" reality and how it works in ways that are acceptable by his peers. He applies what he has discovered in ways that can have a positive or negative impact on society and the planet.

THE CO-CREATIVE SCIENTIST understands that nature comprises the vast and complex reality surrounding him (which he may or may not perceive), and that this reality has order, organization, life vitality and consciousness. He also understands that with consciousness comes intelligence, and that this intelligence offers a broad and unique knowledge from which he can learn. In short, reality teaches the co-creative scientist about reality and how it works. He makes that knowledge useful to others by moving it through his (human) lens, while maintaining respect for and faithfulness to the balance contained within that knowledge. A valid co-creative scientist can only positively impact society and the planet because nature's intelligence always contains inherent balance from the perspective of the immediate issue at hand and the larger picture.

THE CONTEMPORARY SCIENTIST is central to the contemporary scientific process.

THE CO-CREATIVE SCIENTIST functions in full consciousness in connection with nature intelligence, thus creating a partnership with the most qualified expert on the laws of nature and how they apply to reality. This team contains involution/evolution balance because it includes the input of nature (the involution dynamic) and the input of the scientist (the evolution dynamic). It is the co-creative team that is central to co-creative science.

THE CONTEMPORARY SCIENTIFIC METHOD
1. Identify a problem.
2. Observe and collect information relative to the problem.
3. Formulate a hypothesis.
4. Test the hypothesis.

THE CO-CREATIVE SCIENTIFIC METHOD
1 Identify a problem.
2. Create an i/e balanced team with nature that is appropriate for the problem.

3. Verify with nature that what is perceived as a problem by the scientist is indeed being perceived accurately and is something that should be addressed at that time. (This takes into consideration that what humans may perceive as a problem may not, in fact, be a problem from nature's perspective, and to attempt to come up with a "solution" would only result in tampering with balance and the laws of nature, thus creating a real problem.)

4. Understand the problem and collect information relative to it from within the team context. That is, get nature's perspective of the problem and work with nature to obtain whatever education is needed for the scientist to understand the full scope of the problem.

5. Work with nature to create an i/e balanced solution or procedure to address the problem.

6. Set up with nature and test the procedure or solution.

7. Modify and retest the procedure or solution, if necessary, with changes that the scientist and nature consider necessary.

8. Continue to modify and retest, if necessary, until the results indicate to both the scientist and nature that the procedure or solution meets the original goal and maintains full faithfulness to the laws of nature.

9. Apply the results of the testing to the problem within the appropriate larger framework of society and the planet.

10. Educate the public about the solution to this problem, including the laws of nature underlying the solution and how the solution affects them and their lives.

SKILLS NEEDED BY
THE CO-CREATIVE SCIENTIST

If a contemporary scientist decides to take on the training and commit himself to co-creative science, he must discard the inappropriate "habits" he has learned from contemporary science and learn the "habits," skills and attitudes that are essential for co-creative science. He cannot "straddle the fence" by practicing a blend or mixture of contemporary and co-creative science because the two disciplines are mutually exclusive.

This does not mean he must remove himself altogether from the environment of contemporary science in order to function as a co-creative scientist. After all, at the present time, this is where the grants and research funds are. Co-creative science does not require an individual to commit professional suicide. Although someone may presently hold a position in the world of contemporary science, he can still set up and function as a co-creative scientist—especially if he has some autonomy with his research. One of the most convenient aspects about nature intelligence from within the co-creative team is that it is not seen by anyone around the scientist. A co-creative scientist does not walk around with a hairy, strange-looking, cloven-hoofed being by his side that he constantly has to explain to colleagues. ("Oh, him? That's Harry. He's visiting from Ohio. He plays a mean game of poker.") When communicating and consulting with nature, the scientist does not have to say anything aloud. The primary communication bridge with nature intelligence that has been developed at Perelandra does not require audible sound. Therefore, the scientist doesn't even have to move his lips. He need only discipline himself to consult with his partner silently—and then test for nature's input via its answer to a question that has been posed by the scientist. (I describe several communication bridges that have been developed at Perelandra in the next chapter.) What counts in science, as with any profession, is positive, quality results. The co-creative scientist can let his results speak for themselves, and this will be what his colleagues notice. The more success he has in his research, the more his colleagues will notice and acknowledge, and the more they will stand back and "let him do whatever it is that he is doing." He gets all of this without ever uttering a word about "that stuff that he's doing."

Functioning as a co-creative scientist also does not mean that the scientist discards all he has learned through his many years and experiences in contemporary science. He continues to use information from biochemistry, physics, astronomy, geology, etc. when it is appropriate for him to do so, but he uses it within the framework of co-creative science. The knowledge he brings into the partnership becomes part of what he contributes from the perspective of the evolution dynamic. It is a starting point for the scientist. However, when working in partnership with nature, the scientist must be flexible about this starting point and allow for the possibility of nature "showing" him that what he has learned isn't complete or accurate and needs to change in order for him to truly understand the problem and its solution.

The following are the twelve skills required of the co-creative scientist.

1. He must understand his role as a scientist in an i/e balanced team and be able to fully function within this role.

2. He must be willing and able to be educated by nature about reality.

3. He must be skilled in translating information, concepts and insight from beyond his range of normal sensory perception into that range without compromising the integrity, balance and intent of the information. He must then be able to communicate this information to the people who will ultimately benefit from or be changed by the information, concepts and insight.

4. He must know how to ask nature simple, clear, accurate questions that are worded with the intent to discover truth and not for the purpose of proving his own theories. And he must know how to ask questions about things he cannot presently perceive.

5. He must be willing and able to move forward into the "unknown," trusting that nature knows what it is doing and where it is going.

6. He must be able to observe well, process and absorb experience fully, and learn the new without tying it to the intellectual frameworks he previously knew.

7. He must know when it is appropriate to suspend his intellect and how to do this.

8. He must understand intellect, intent and intuition in their various functions and be skilled in those functions.

9. He must understand that the sum total of his own knowledge is no more than a tiny drop in the bucket when compared to the knowledge that exists in reality and with nature.

10. He must use co-creative science in his daily life, not because he feels "required" to do so, but because he knows that

this science is not something to be used solely in a scientific laboratory.

11. He must know how to think with his heart, as well as his head, and with the intent to discover truth.

12. He must have a balanced sense of ego and self-worth, and a personal commitment to honesty and overall integrity in his scientific work and his life in general. If he has an inflated ego, he will have the tendency to take charge in the partnership and relegate nature to the position of a partner only when it is convenient for the scientist. When this occurs, nature will not fight him and will simply "step back" until he "comes to his senses" and once again establishes a peer relationship with nature. If his ego is "under inflated," he will feel overwhelmed by the scope of what nature knows and be reluctant to function well or hold up his end of the i/e balanced partnership. In this situation, nature will automatically adjust its input to reflect the reduced input of the scientist and the partnership will not be able to grow or meet its potential. It will do this because nature inherently functions *in balance* and will not "overpower" the partnership by giving more information and insight than the scientist can handle. In other words, nature does not respond beyond that which is initiated and set by the human who represents the evolution dynamic in i/e balance. To do so would create i/e *imbalance*. To establish and maintain balance, nature must respond to an individual in kind. In short, there is balance within i/e balance.

4

The Making of a Co-Creative Scientist

I F YOU LOOK AROUND, YOU'LL probably notice that there are no colleges or universities where someone may go to receive a degree in co-creative science. Actually, the vast majority of educational facilities have never heard the term "co-creative science." (There have been a handful of classes that teach co-creative science in philosophy and environmental studies.) But even without the support of a formal educational system, you can enter your own program that will result in all the education and training required for practicing co-creative science. Until contemporary scientists see (and admit that they see) the results that demonstrate that this new science is extraordinarily effective in every way and that it addresses the serious situations we face, and soften their objections, prejudices, fear and general resistance about anything as new and different as this, a co-creative scientist desiring to work within the normal scientific community will also have to obtain the credentials in his field of interest that are required by that community. Which credentials you obtain first—those in contemporary science or those in co-creative science—is up to you. My suggestion is that you follow your gut instinct in this matter. My personal choice would be to get the credentials in contemporary science first and get that out of the way. But this would be my choice. I do not recommend that you enter both programs simultaneously. The two sciences are too different, and I suspect that you would feel like you were trying to balance two different worlds. To put it mildly, this could be frustrating and stressful. One other point about the two sciences: No matter how impressive the credentials are for a contemporary scientist, he cannot "roll over" those credentials and apply them to co-creative science. In co-creative science, he starts with a clean slate.

If you should choose to get your credentials in co-creative science first—the requirements for the credentials in co-creative science are explained at the end of this chapter—you might discover that you will not want to work as a scientist in the world of contemporary science and take your chances operating as an "independent." I do not have contemporary science credentials. But I do meet all the requirements needed for the co-creative scientist—and I function as an "independent." That is, I don't address contemporary science, its requirements, structure or financial benefits at all. I work within an environment that is set up solely for co-creative science. My work is self-supporting, so I have no need to look for funding or grants. Consequently, I also have no one looking over my shoulder telling me what to do. I work on issues and problems using the co-creative scientific method as described in Chapter 3. As processes and programs for addressing problems are formulated and tested, and they meet the high standards set by both nature and me, I publish the information. This allows anyone who is interested in trying something new and effective the chance to do just that. Many thousands of people now work with the different health and environmental programs that have been developed at Perelandra and have experienced tremendous success in using them. Their lives and the condition of the environment around them have improved dramatically. To me, this is what science is all about.

When I "entered" the world of co-creative science in 1977, there were no books about how to do anything practical in partnership with nature. There were just a handful of books introducing the concept of a nature intelligence with which you could communicate. That is where I got my first clue about this area of nature. I read two books about the Findhorn garden that was growing in sand in Findhorn, Scotland, and about how the people who started that garden worked with nature intelligences. Immediately, everything in these two books rang true for me—despite the fact that what I was reading was absolutely crazy—and I received the encouragement I needed to open to a new world. Today, as a result of the research with nature going on at Perelandra, we have a number of books and papers that give insight about what it's like to work in this partnership—from both the human perspective and nature's perspective—and that give step-by-step instructions on what you need to do in order to work in conjunction with nature to address specific environmental and health issues. These books and papers are the course material for someone entering the "school of co-creative science." There is actually a lot of material, and a great deal can be learned if you carefully study the information and work with the various processes and programs. This alone may take you three or more years before you will feel you are familiar and comfortable with everything that is published.

However, if you take three, even four, years to diligently study this information and learn to use the processes and programs in your life and immediate environment, you still will not have met the requirements to be a co-creative scientist. You will have become an exceptionally well-informed individual who chooses to integrate co-creative science into his life. (I might add here that this kind of diligent studying is not required for someone who chooses to integrate this science into his daily life. Many thousands of people get one book, read it and jump right into using the program or process that is described. In fact, this is the usual way someone begins working with co-creative science. And they receive excellent results. I am only saying that no matter how much a person studies the Perelandra material and works with the processes, he is *not* a co-creative scientist.)

What makes the education of the co-creative scientist unique is the classroom you must enter into with nature. The books and processes lay one foundation for you. But the classroom with nature gives you the real foundation of the co-creative scientist. In this classroom, you "allow" nature to function as your teacher. It is a critical time when the two members of the team get to know one another and the foundation for the i/e partnership in science is formed. You become familiar with the range and depth of nature's knowledge and its intellectual properties that function so differently from ours. I recently asked nature if an estimated time could be given for someone entering this kind of classroom with the intent of becoming a co-creative scientist. The answer: about four years. I was in class with nature for seven years—but I didn't have any texts to study that could have shortened the time needed for a full education. When I say that I was in class for seven years, I mean that for seven years I presented myself as the student and looked to nature as my teacher. The class is completely experiential. You don't sit in a classroom, take notes, pass tests and write a paper. You learn through experience. Nature sets the pace and subject matter in light of who you, the student, are and how much you are able to absorb. In short, the course is completely designed by nature especially for you. As you move through it, you learn to see reality from nature's perspective.

It is a deeply personal experience and unlike any class situation you will ever have gone through. And it can be tough because it is not always easy to let go of what we assume to be true about life and reality, despite the evidence to the contrary that we are experiencing. It takes time (three years of study plus four years of class or four or five years of combined study and class) because our framework of logic must change. Co-creative science is not built on your old logic or the logic that is the foundation for contemporary science. It is a new way of experiencing and responding to life and life's problems.

My classroom was a vegetable garden. I'd like to say that I was smart enough at the time to deliberately choose this classroom, but I didn't have a clue about what I was doing. I only knew I was to do it. I had been gardening for three years prior to entering the classroom. In those three years, I had shifted my approach from traditional gardening complete with chemical pesticides to organic gardening methods. It was my frustration about the plethora of advice one receives just to do one simple task in organic gardening that convinced me, once I read the two Findhorn books, that what we really needed to do was ignore everyone's advice and ask nature directly about what to do. Consequently, once I read those two books, my attention immediately turned to my vegetable garden. And this is how the first co-creative science classroom was chosen. Luckily, it could not have been a better choice. I feel certain that I was able to rivet my focus on the garden so easily because nature was also "pushing" me in that direction. It was a perfect co-creative science classroom.

I entered the class knowing with every fiber of my being that, despite everything I had learned about gardening the previous three years, I knew nothing. I now made no decisions about what went into the garden, where plants were to be placed, or how to maintain the garden. Nature was completely in charge of the classroom. And, over the seven years, I did not initiate any projects. To do so would have placed me in the position of a peer with nature. Instead, I "stepped back" and let nature take the lead. By the time I took on the role of peer with nature in science, I had a deep understanding of who my partner was, what my partner knew, what my role was, who I was, and an understanding of reality and how it works as seen from my partner's "eyes." When I initiated the first project, I also instinctively knew when and how to "stand back" and let my partner take the lead on something I initiate.

This is needed when it is important for the scientist to resume the role of the student and let nature teach him how to accurately perceive something new and understand what he is perceiving in order to proceed together as a team toward a common solution or goal. In short, although I left the classroom nearly fourteen years ago, I have never stopped being the student. By the time I was ready to take on the responsibilities and role of peer with nature in science, I knew that my education had just begun, but now I was qualified to continue that education from within the framework of the co-creative science partnership.

To help you understand the classroom concept, I'm presenting my first-year class. I have written about this first-year co-creative garden in the book *Behaving as if the God in All Life Mattered*. But for *Co-Creative Science*, I want to present that year again—this time through the lens of a co-creative science student in the classroom with nature. I describe the details of this year as I did in *Behaving*, but this time I have inserted comments and explanations from the perspective of the student and the scientist.

I entered the classroom with three important communication skills. Since I had no books for getting any practical information about working with nature intelligence, I needed to have the ability to communicate with nature already in place before I started the class. If you wish, you can learn these skills after you enter the classroom because what you need for bridging the communication gap with nature is now published and ready for you. Prior to 1976, I had spent several years exploring different aspects of meditation. From this work, I learned a self-testing kinesiology technique. (You may learn this skill for yourself. The testing technique is described in the appendix.) Kinesiology is an impressive sounding word for muscle testing. Chiropractors and other health-care practitioners have used it for years as a diagnostic tool. However, I had not yet been exposed to this tool as it is used in health-care and learned the technique for myself from my earlier meditation work.

This work also taught me the discipline needed for developing my sensory system so that I could do what I call "translation." I will explain that further because the nature sessions that are included in *Co-Creative Science* are a result of this working process between nature and myself. When I translate information from nature, I am in full control of my consciousness. I connect with the nature intelligence in much the same manner as two people connect via a phone line. Nature then directs information to me about a subject in the form of energy—words, visualizations, insights and concepts without sound. My job as translator is to assign to the specific impulses of energy the words that most fully carry the intent of the energy that was directed to me. To understand this process more easily, just think of the job of the United Nations interpreters. They don't go into a trance state when they work. They develop the art of focused listening and the ability to translate intent, thought, expression and concept from one language pattern to another. If you take away the audible sounds and have only the projection to the translator of the energy patterns behind the sound, you have a good idea of the process I work with: communication in the form of energy. I just translate that communication into the words that are faithful to the intent and expression of the energy I experience. And very like the U.N. interpreter, I am only as good at this as my innate ability combined with training, discipline, care and a lot of years of experience.

At the time that I was first developing these communication skills, I didn't know I would be using them as a bridge to nature intelligence. In fact, I didn't even know about nature intelligence at the time. You may never develop an ability to translate. It will depend on what skills are appropriate for you. However, to blaze this trail with nature, it was useful for me to have this particular skill. But to function fully as a co-creative scientist, you only need to develop kinesiology and sharpen your intuition. The two, when used together, are all that is needed between you and nature.

I also entered my classroom with a strong gut feeling that was based on something I was experiencing at the time. In 1973, my partner Clarence and I moved from Washington, D.C., to the land we named "Perelandra." It was originally ten acres of woods situated in Virginia farm country. Clarence was working for the Xerox Corporation and had to commute about fifty-five miles each way. Besides gardening, I concentrated my days on the new land, cleaning up the damage that had been created when our house was built. Because Clarence was gone for so many hours during the day, I spent most of my time alone on the land. I loved it. But I sometimes felt an unexplainable heightening of energy from the woods—especially in the evening. I didn't feel threatened by it. In fact, I figured that once I settled down and got used to the silence, I wouldn't feel these sensations. In short, I assumed it was all coming from my head. When I read the two Findhorn books,

I knew immediately that this "nature thing" was what I was feeling from the woods. It was pure gut instinct. Granted, it was a huge leap from a sensation that could be explained away by any half-decent psychologist to a nature intelligence that was capable of communication. But I think gut instincts are often not logical and are just what is needed to move us in an entirely new direction. I *knew* that the sensations I was picking up weren't coming from my head, and that this new nature information was my key to discovery. It was at this point that I entered the classroom.

As you read about this first year, notice how the classes began gently, simply and, as I learned more, how they gradually intensified. NOTE: How I describe these events is primarily from the perspective of the first-year student. Throughout, I have interspersed comments written from the perspective of the scientist reviewing this experience twenty years after it occurred.

MY FIRST YEAR IN CLASS WITH NATURE

One evening in early January 1977, just after reading the Findhorn books, I walked into the woods and announced in a loud, clear voice, "I want to do at Perelandra what they did at Findhorn. I want to work with devas and I want to work with nature spirits. I invite all of you to make yourselves known to me. I am ready to learn from you."

Then I left the woods, returned to the house, sat quietly and waited.

In *Behaving*, I describe this moment as a ceremony, and it was. But from the perspective of the co-creative science student, it was the moment I stated my intent to learn from nature. This is vital for the student to do. Nature will not start functioning as a teacher unless you specifically state that you want it to. My statement was simple and rather open-ended. I used the terms "deva" and "nature spirit" because that was the terminology I had just learned from the Findhorn books. I then sealed my stated intent by physically acting on it—by sitting quietly and opening myself to whatever was to happen next. From the moment I verbalized this statement, my garden ceased being a vegetable garden. It became a co-creative science classroom that was utilizing the structure of a vegetable garden as its focus. (At the end of this chapter, I present a guideline for opening such a classroom and suggestions about how to make your initial statement of intent in a clear and concise way.)

The response that I got from nature was immediate. In fact, I had the same experience that Dorothy Maclean had at Findhorn when she first connected with devas. I had a "crowd of voices" coming at me, all talking at the same time—all telling me that it was "about time." I connected with them and found that they had been waiting for this for some time. I remembered that in the Findhorn book, when Dorothy described this experience, she said she simply asked the devas to speak to her one at a time. Having nothing to lose, I tried the same thing. Much to my amazement, they responded instantaneously. And from that point on, I clearly heard one devic voice at a time.

A NOTE: In the early years of my classroom, I experienced nature intelligence as a collection of different and distinct energies. In a sense, this is an accurate description. But I did not yet have a sense of one massive intelligence for nature, as described in Chapter 2, that is made up of countless elements of knowledge that constitute the vast devic and nature spirit levels of operation. I only sensed all the differentiation. Consequently, I referred to these two levels of intelligence in more individualistic terms: the devas, a nature spirit and so forth. In actuality, I still will use this language today, only now I understand more clearly what I mean when I use it.

The following is how I described "deva" in *Behaving.*

Deva (pronounced: day'-vah) is the Sanskrit word for "body of light." I found the devic level to be a level of consciousness very high in vibration. It's as if someone were to hit a bunch of tuning forks and we could distinguish the vibratory difference between them rather than the sound difference. I found the devic vibration to feel extremely high and light. It did not even resemble anything I had experienced in meditation previously. Its essence was clearly different.

The word "architect" has been used by others when describing what devas do—and I, also, find this to be the most appropriate word. For example, it is the devic level that designs the blueprint and draws together all the various energies that make up the complex "package" for the carrot. The Carrot Deva "pulls together" the various energies that determine the size, color, texture, taste, nutritional needs, growing season, shape, flower and seed process of the carrot. In essence, the Deva of the Carrot is responsible for the carrot's entire physical package. It maintains the vision—that is, the complete reality—of the carrot in perfection and holds that collection of energies together in their unique pattern as it passes from one vibratory level to another on its route to becoming physical to the five senses. Everything about the carrot on a practical level, as well as on the more expanded, universal level, is known by the Carrot Deva.

Each day I would sit in the garden, become quietly focused and connect with the devic level. A deva would come into my awareness and identify itself. I was then given instructions. I was told what seeds to buy, what fertilizer to use, how far apart to plant the seeds, when to thin the plants and how much space to leave between them, spacing between the rows, desired amount of sunlight, and so on.

As each deva came into my awareness, I noticed that there was a slight shift in vibration, that each had its own vibration. After awhile, I could recognize which deva was entering my awareness. This led me to develop the ability to call upon specific devas by "aiming" my awareness for the deva's own vibratory pattern. It was as if I was faced with a gigantic telephone system and I had to learn how to make all the different connections. Then I was able to make calls in as well as receive calls.

(Later in the summer, I discovered that all I had to do to connect with a specific deva was to simply request the connection. For example, to connect with the Deva of the Carrot, I only needed to say, "I'd like to be connected with the Deva of the Carrot." Immediately I'd feel the familiar vibration of the Carrot Deva in my awareness. I knew the connection had been made and we were ready to work together. This connection business couldn't have been more simple.)

One day, I felt a very different, more expansive vibration and found myself connected to the Overlighting Deva of the Garden. This deva talked about such things as the overall layout of the garden, its timing, its progression and its shape. From it, I was also told to change my gardening method to the mulch method—a method whereby six inches of hay, grass clippings and leaves are kept on the garden at all times. Two years later, I was told to switch from the traditional straight rows to a garden of concentric circles.

After a somewhat lengthy session with the Overlighting Deva of the Garden, I was contacted by the Soil Deva and given information about soil that dovetailed with what I had received from the Overlighting Deva.

The rhythm of one deva after another contacting me continued throughout that spring and early summer. I wasn't given the "full scoop" on any one subject. Rather, I received just what I needed for what I was to act on at that moment. Then, at a later time, I got more information. After each session, I jotted down in a notebook what information had been given to me, either practically or as an insight about what I was doing and why. Then, as soon as I could, I acted on anything that needed doing.

From the perspective of the student, it is absolutely critical that we constantly work with nature's lessons in action. I'd get an insight or I'd hear something specific about the thing that I was looking at or working on. I didn't get information about something I was going to need to do next week. Everything was in the moment. And I would then act on the basis of the information I had gotten. I didn't just sit on it. A co-creative science student does not sit around with information and say, "Oh, isn't this interesting." He acts on that new information and observes the results. If no changes can be observed, he continues to watch as whatever he was working on moves through its cycle. At some point, he will observe a change that will be directly attributable to the action he took that was based on the new information. At this point, he will begin to understand something about the underlying principle of the original insight and action.

To give you an idea of the kind of information that comes from the devic level, I share with you two examples of sessions I translated. I had this first session on March 22, 1977, during that first-year garden. I had the second session on January, 1990, nearly thirteen years later. I have chosen these two examples because I want you to see that working with nature in partnership is a learning process and not a magical, already-developed gift. This is why you are in the classroom. When you begin, communication is simple and you do not feel overwhelmed by the information. As time goes on, your abilities improve and the depth of your communication with nature improves in kind. Also notice how the language used in the two sessions changed, as well.

OVERLIGHTING DEVA OF
THE PERELANDRA GARDEN

1977: *We urge you to join our creative process. When you plant a seed, invoke the deva and nature spirits connected with that seed. The seed is the door between you and the various energies that are drawn together on the devic level and cared for by the nature spirits. Once you have planted the seed, put out the call for the deva to draw together all the individual energy components of that variety. Ask that the nature spirits receive the energies and, in essence, fuse them to the seed. The seed contains the potential of the plant's perfection. The grounding of the plant's energy into the seed activates that potential and transforms it into full physical reality. As you call the energy into five-senses form, see its energy channel touch the seed as it is grounded by the nature spirits.*

By joining in our creative process in this manner, you will begin to see the importance of working with the nature energies with clarity. We urge you to plant the garden in this new way and see the difference your clear participation as a co-creative partner with us makes in the germination of the seeds and the quality of plant growth.

The second session is on geopathic zones—that is, well-defined and detectable energy realities within an area's soil, water or air. They can sometimes cause distress or illness to a person who lives or works in a zone-impacted area. I first heard about geopathic zones in 1989. There is considerable information about their effects, primarily in the area of health. Researchers have found people living in the same area and having the same illness. Further research then showed that these people were all living on a geopathic zone. For example, some people with insomnia slept in beds located above geopathic zones. To understand geopathic zones better, I asked nature for information.

THE DEVA OF GEOPATHIC ZONES

1990: Geopathic zones are self-contained energy realities found in the planet's soil, water or air that can either enhance the health, balance and well-being of any life systems that come into contact with them or adversely impact, even destroy, some life systems that are impacted by them. In recent years, humans have become more aware of geopathic zones because of the detrimental impact these zones have had on those living within a zone area. The impact may range from mild discomfort, sleep difficulties and constant but mild illnesses to chronic, life-threatening conditions.

But geopathic zones are complex and cannot be adequately covered in one short definition. Therefore, they should not be looked at solely as mysterious life-threatening forces. What have been referred to as "geopathic zones" do not always originate from the same circumstances nor do they function with the same dynamics. Geopathic zones can refer to a soil/earth phenomenon, a rock-vein phenomenon, a waterway phenomenon or an atmospheric phenomenon. They may consist of any one of these or include a combination of several in order to create a larger, more complex geopathic zone.

In order to understand how geopathic zones form, one must look at them from two separate perspectives: the human perspective and the nature perspective. Let us address the nature perspective first. If one were to view the planet without human habitation, one would see a nature-dominant planet in which cycles, rhythms, patterns and movement play out in an unrestricted, natural way. In this environment, elements of the planet—the elements comprising the soil and its core, those elements that are a part of the planet's surface, and the elements comprising the atmosphere—would shift and move as part of the planet's natural patterns. We point this out to you to emphasize that one cannot say that geopathic zones are created solely by humans and are caused by adverse human impact on the planet. This is not true. Left on its own, the natural rhythm of the planet would include a natural movement and shifting of its elements in such a way as to create a physical environment that humans call "geopathic zones."

These zones may be seen as veins, as broad areas, as circles and as wide swaths narrowing into thinner swaths. They may occur above ground, on the surface or below ground. Their depth varies as much as their width. From the broadest perspective, they are a concentration of "like" matter . . . like attracting like—for it is the natural magnetic phenomenon of horizontal compatibility occurring between elements on all levels that creates the kinds of zones of which we now speak. As the earth's elements shift and move, you will find that the key to understanding this movement is horizontal compatibility: like moving into the direction and vicinity of like.

The result is the creation of compatible environments. (You keep seeing a field of wildflowers. This picture is from us.) Using that field of wildflowers as an example, we of nature would say that this is a perfect visual example of horizontal compatibility. Now, many humans would look at such a field and say that the wildflowers that grow there do so because the physical conditions are correct for supporting their growth. And that the wildflowers that do not grow in the field are absent because the physical conditions do not support their growth. We of nature look at the field and say it is a compatible environment created by the natural magnetic attraction of horizontally compatible elements, including those wildflowers. As an environment, it excludes nothing. From our point of view, this is a geopathic zone and can be defined in size and scope by the compatible elements growing in the zone and supported by that zone.

We use the imagery of the wildflower field purposely. Many feel that geopathic zones are, by definition, "negative." Often this is because geopathic zones can be powerful in terms of an energy dynamic—the sum being greater and more powerful than its parts. Also, these zones can feel exceptionally powerful to humans because the parts or elements in a specific zone may be, in and of themselves, especially powerful. Some zones create and emit an energy that can be described as gentle, some soft, others strong, and still others powerful beyond that which some humans can endure.

Now, add humans to the planet. If given total freedom, humans would automatically shift and move around the planet in response to the natural earth shifts that are occurring. The human soul and body would seek a compatible environment. We include the human soul because the body, although comprised of nature, is shaped and molded by the individual's soul. Consequently, humans would seek horizontal compatibility as a unit.

Let us, at this point, address the geopathic zones that adversely impact and cause problems to humans. Like attracts like. That which the human creates and releases in the planet adds to and becomes a part of that which defines the planet. Nothing magically disappears. Another way of saying this is that nothing dies. That which is in mass form becomes a part of the environment on which it sits. Feelings and emotions as energy have a more ebb-and-flow dynamic to them. Several things can occur with feelings and emotions. One is that, once emitted, they will become a part of the environment in which they were emitted. If the emotions were expressed and resolved in a complete and balanced manner, they will become a part of that environment as an element already in balance. If the emotions were not "grounded" and therefore not resolved, they will become a part of that environment as an unbalanced element. If allowed to remain as part of the environment, as has been the case with most emotional input throughout the planet, those emotions will impact everything else that is part of the environment and initiate a movement of accommodation of the environmental elements toward the unbalanced emotion. In short, the molecules comprising the environment in which the ungrounded emotions are impacting will change. And because of horizontal compatibility, any elements that were part of a heretofore balanced environment that cannot make the molecular changes required to enfold the new unbalanced emotional element will move out of that environment, first in energy and then followed by form, to a more compatible environment.

As molecules within an environment alter to accommodate the emotional input, that environment attracts to it a different range of elements. There is a new horizontal compatibility. This is what you refer to as an "emotional sinkhole." The new environment will also naturally attract to it humans who are comfortable with the range and quality of emotions supported by it. Often, once imbalance becomes integrated into an environment, it encourages even greater imbalance. This may appear to contradict "like attracting like" or horizontal compatibility. But one of the dynamics of imbalance is that it encourages an intensification of the problem. Conversely, one of

the dynamics of balance is that it encourages an intensi-
fication of balance as well as the corresponding movement
forward to a new level of balance. So, in terms of the environ-
ment that is now not in balance, you have a downspiraling
effect that was initiated by humans through their release of
unbalanced emotional energy. The initial imbalance as well
as the downspiraling effect are both initiated by humans. Na-
ture does not have as part of its makeup the mechanism that
would create and initiate an emotional downspiral.

Let us give you an example of geopathic zones. We will ad-
dress a small urban row house that is sitting on one larger
geopathic zone that has as part of its makeup several inter-
secting line-like zones. These are several "environments" that
are complete within themselves and are related to one an-
other in terms of compatibility. The occupants have detected
two line-like zones by using dowsing techniques. However,
there are in actuality five more intersecting line-like zones
moving through their property and house. You will find that
in heavily populated areas, where humans and nature have
had high impact, the frequency of geopathic zones will in-
crease considerably.

Now what is occurring in this home is an example of how
humans, using free will and strength in determination, can
stop an environmental geopathic downspiral. These occupants
are not people who have naturally gravitated to an environ-
ment in which they are completely comfortable. They have ex-
ercised free will and taken on an environment that, in some
ways (and not all), is uncomfortable—and they have moved
to change it. This same phenomenon occurs in urban areas
that are going through renovation and renewal. New people

deliberately choose to move in with the intent to revitalize and change an area. In our example, the two line-like zones that were detected were the two zones that were most out of balance with the occupants. They detected the zones because of an especially strong electrical charge that was being set up due to difference; that is, the people living there were so different in makeup from the two line zones that an especially charged electrical field had developed between them and the zones, making detection not only possible but essential. For the health and well-being of the occupants, the geopathic zones needed to be addressed.

When working with geopathic zones, the intent is to return the zone(s) to a strong environmental balance. Those elements in the zone that do not reflect the new balance will be automatically released to continue on an evolutionary path (as is the case of emotional energy), or will shift to another more compatible zone (as in the case of nature and mass).

Nature then went on to give me the setup and steps for the Geopathic Zone Process. We tested these steps and published them in the *Perelandra Garden Workbook II* in 1990.

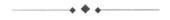

1977: Just about every evening during the early months of my first year in nature's classroom, I would tell Clarence about what I had learned from the devic level that day. From the very beginning, the concept of there being intelligence within nature made sense to him.

One evening as I was chattering on about devas, an arc of light came into my visual awareness. Clarence was sitting across the room in a rocker facing me, and just off to his left was the arc, about four feet high, four inches wide, the shape of a new moon. At first I thought my mind was playing tricks on me. After all, it was late in the evening. I tried to narrow my focus more on Clarence's face in an attempt not to let this "thing" disturb me. But it kept pulsating light at me. Finally, I laughed, admitted defeat to myself, and told Clarence that there was no way I could continue this conversation with this thing pulsating at me. Then I described what I was seeing. He said he had been feeling a presence next to him but couldn't see anything. Quite frankly, I didn't know what to do with the thing. So I offered it a cup of tea! The thing pulsated even brighter at me. I closed my eyes, first the right, then the left, to see if by chance a piece of lint on my eyeball was causing this strange sight. My eyes were clean. Clarence left the room to make tea—for the two of us, not for our guest—and while he was out, I gave my full attention over to the arc of light. It got brighter still, and, with great gentleness, a sense of awareness washed through me. The light's energy was touching into me. It identified itself as a deva and said it was there to show me that devas were a reality.

This was the moment when the devic level of nature intelligence and I formally and "officially" made our connection. When Clarence returned with our tea, we continued our discussion with the deva still off to his left. As we talked, the arc of light slowly removed itself from my awareness and was no longer visible.

You have probably noted that this event occurred outside the garden classroom. Although we had set up the formal classroom, it was not unusual for nature to project insight or an experience, as was the case this time, when I least expected it. It didn't take me long to realize that some lessons worked best with the surprise element added and would occur when I was in my most relaxed state. When something like this happened, I was instructed by nature to "bring it up" in class the next day. I would describe what I saw or heard and what I understood about the experience. That way, nature could gauge what I was perceiving from experiences it was giving me.

In February, I was told to go into the woods at midnight to a specific white oak tree. I was to sit by the tree and lean my back against it. There was snow on the ground and a biting wind was making it icy cold, but I bundled up and trudged out to the oak tree. I set a stool next to the trunk, and I leaned my back against the tree.

In less than a minute, I felt a strange energy from the tree flow into my back. My body began to fill, so to keep things from getting "crowded," I decided to use my breath to flow my own energy into the tree. It was a pleasurable sensation —comforting, supportive and stabilizing. My body got so warm that when I returned to the tree the next night at midnight as instructed, I didn't bother wearing a coat.

I continued this routine for about two weeks. Then I was told to stop.

During the same period, we were running low on wood for our stove, and Clarence had to find some suitable trees to cut for our supply. I was told by the Deva of the Woods where there stood a dead, perfectly seasoned thirty-foot tree that would be ideal for our needs. I was also told that we would have to enlist the help of the nature spirits in order to get the tree down without doing a lot of damage.

Sure enough, there was the tree, deep in the woods. It was leaning, which meant that the angle of the fall was limited to that one direction. If the tree fell exactly straight, it would do no damage. If it fell no more than two inches to the left or right from this straight line, it would damage a number of healthy trees.

I talked to Clarence about what I was learning concerning the role of nature spirits. I suggested that when he was ready to fell the tree, he verbalized his request to the nature spirits for their help in the process. I told him to state very clearly what he wanted to have happen with the tree and how he wanted it to fall.

Early one morning, Clarence headed for the tree. I was just waking up when I heard a tremendous shout from him, "No! No! Four feet to the left!" About two seconds later, there was a crash that shook the house. A few seconds after that, I felt myself being kissed gently on the forehead. A clear, precise kiss. No mistaking it for a fly, or the wind. Then I heard a voice tell me that we had "passed the test," the test with the tree, and I was now formally connected with the nature spirit level of intelligence at Perelandra. My energy experience with the oak tree had been my preparation for this moment. The bearer of the kiss was a nature spirit.

(This kiss and the arc of light are examples of what nature talked about in Chapter 2 when defining nature intelligence and how special communication bridges can be instantaneously set up by nature for special moments with us.)

Clarence came into the bedroom with a stunned look on his face and explained what had happened with the tree. He asked for the nature spirits' help just as I had suggested, then sawed the tree as carefully as he could so it would fall properly. As it came down through the air, he saw that it was falling way off course—in fact, it was falling four feet off to the right. Because of our conversations about nature, he had become so convinced of the reality of nature spirits that when faced with this crisis his knee-jerk reaction was to shout to them exactly what needed to happen. In mid-air, the thirty-foot tree moved four feet to the left and came down exactly on target.

In *Behaving*, I refer to nature spirits as "blue-collar workers" and describe them and their work as follows.

The devas create the package that includes the different components of a plant. Once the "package" of energy is formed, the devas then "hold" the package together as it "travels" from one level to another, changing and adjusting its vibration as it acclimates to the Earth's reality. Once the package begins to take on five-senses form, the nature spirits take over. It is the responsibility of the nature spirits not only to receive the package of energy but to stabilize its fusion into its proper form as well. In short, they maintain a plant's light, its essence, its life pattern and cycles.

Devas are universal in dynamic. My Deva of the Carrot is the same as your Deva of the Carrot. But nature spirits are regional. My nature spirits at Perelandra are not the same as those working around you in your area.

Nature spirits, like devas, can also appear as bodies of light energy. But their vibration feels more dense than the devic vibration does. It is still a very profound experience for us to feel. If we could add sound to these different nature spirit vibrations, we would hear clear, high-pitched, pleasing, pure tones—beautiful high notes with soft, distinctive vibratos. By comparison, devic notes would sound even higher in tone, but equally distinctive, pleasing and pure.

Over the years when I've talked about these things with others, many people have said to me that they have had devic experiences—profound, pure experiences. As we talked about it more, I realized that they actually experienced the nature spirit level and thought it was the devic level because they didn't expect such a high sensation from nature spirits. For some reason, some people believe that nature spirits are "lower" in some imagined hierarchy than devas. Perhaps even I am fueling this belief by referring to one as "architect" and the other as "blue-collar worker." I don't mean for these tags to imply hierarchy. (Just as when referring to humans they shouldn't imply hierarchy.) They are both equal components of nature intelligence. It's only that they have very different job descriptions.

Nature spirits are the implementors. They are responsible for tending to the well-being of all form, and they ensure that the devic rhythms and patterns that create a full life cycle are activated and maintained. To do this, nature spirits "read" the devic information and ensure that this information is fully implemented into action. They also maintain a quality of fusion between the form and the life energies contained within that form. If I were to desire a change in the color of the carrot, I would seek that change on the devic level. That is part of the architectural package of the carrot. However, if I wish to prepare the soil, know the best times for watering the plants and how much to water, I would look to the nature spirit level for help because I'm now focused on the day-to-day issues of the carrot's life cycle.

I had read that at Findhorn there was an area set aside specifically for the use of nature spirits. It was a place where humans didn't enter and it was left wild. I felt that I should do the same at Perelandra. So I picked a spot on the edge of the woods next to the garden and roped it off as a gesture, designating the area to be exclusively for nature spirits. After roping it off, I stood in the middle of the area and invited the nature spirits to come to this special place that I called the "Elemental Annex." Immediately, a great rush of energy streamed in and I heard, "Finally! Now we can get down to business!" Feeling very much out of place, I gingerly stepped out of the area. The Elemental Annex then became the base of operations for the Perelandra nature spirits.

This is one time I actually initiated an action or activity in the classroom. It was appropriate for me to do this because a nature spirit sanctuary is a gift from a human to nature. It must be initiated by us. My experience with the Elemental Annex verified to me that nature had enthusiastically accepted my gift and my gesture.

Thanks to centuries of tradition, fairy tales and folklore, most people think of nature spirits in terms of elves, gnomes, fairies—the "little people" of the woods. I have experienced nature spirits as swirling spheres of light energy. I have walked through the woods with one of these "balls of energy" moving beside me, and, when necessary, I've moved around a tree while the "ball of energy" continued to move straight through the tree, coming out the other side. My personal inner vision lies in the area of energy. I tend to see waves of energy, energy dynamics and interplay; in fact, I tend to see the reality around me as energy first, then five-senses form. So I'm comfortable with the concept of an energy reality. I was not familiar with or comfortable with the concept of fairies, elves and gnomes. I simply didn't have a background steeped in fairy tales and folklore. So out of consideration for me, when this level of nature intelligence chose to be visible, it chose a context with which I was comfortable—energy. Had I seen an elf or a gnome come toward me, I definitely would have checked myself into a rubber room.

I have also learned from the nature spirits that they do indeed appear to humans in the form of elves, fairies, gnomes, and so forth, but only to people who are comfortable with these concepts. To do this, they make use of our own thought forms. We humans have developed a long tradition of what, for example, an elf looks like. We have books and stories and artists' conceptions, all detailing the little creatures. Those highly stylized thought forms are released from us and become part of the Earth's reality. When a nature spirit desires to become visible to someone, it has access to this reality and can use these thought forms or combinations of thought forms to aid it in creating a "body" through which to appear. So it is quite possible for someone who has actually seen nature spirits to interpret it as seeing elves.

But there is a reverse side that comes into play here. I've met people who say they've seen nature spirits. When I've talked to them about the interaction that took place between them during those experiences, I've realized that they weren't seeing true nature spirits. The key here is that man cannot will a nature spirit to appear to him. But some people want to see them so badly, they actually create their own animated thought form. It's visible. It moves. It talks to them. But it is their own creation and its words are their own thoughts that are being projected through this creation. Most of the time, it makes the person involved feel uncomfortable. And that's the other key. Dynamics of love and balance constantly flow from the nature spirit level. In my many years of working with this level directly, I've never felt fear or apprehension. I've always felt balance, protection, consideration and care directed to me.

We humans have barely begun to understand the power we have. We don't realize that out of our own desire, an intense desire, we can create moving thought form. And since these things are our own creation, we give them all their characteristics—even their emotional characteristics. So if we think elves can be mean, we'll create a mean elf. This thought form then becomes frightening to us.

Nature spirits have taken a lot of "bad raps" because of our mistaking our own thought forms for them. They are part of the guardianship of life on Earth. They deal with life forces constantly. They're not in the business of negating life. And it's not part of their makeup to provoke fear in us.

One other thing about nature spirits: they are an extremely powerful level of nature intelligence. They are responsible for the existence of all form around us, and at the blink of a flea's eye, they can remove that form. They are many things, but they are never, *never* cute. Nor are they ever controlled by us. They seek a co-creative partnership with humans, and they are in the position to accept nothing less.

In February, I was given the layout of the garden. Starting at one end, I paced off the rows according to what I was receiving from the devic level. Wherever I was told there was to be a row, I put a stake in the ground, labeling on it what I was told was to be planted there. In previous years, it took me a full day to complete this chore. With help from nature, the process took about a half hour.

I started some seeds in flats in the house—tomatoes, green peppers, broccoli, cabbage, Brussels sprouts and cauliflower. I planted each vegetable according to the instructions I was getting. Then I called on the deva and nature spirits connected with the vegetable to ground or fuse its energies into the seed. The response was astounding. Nothing took more than two days to germinate. The tomatoes germinated and had their first set of leaves in less than two days. The seedlings then grew twice as fast as normal. The quality of color in the plants was vibrant. There is a difference in the shade of green between broccoli, cabbage, Brussels sprouts and cauliflower. Now these differences were crystal clear. When I touched the plants, the leaves had a different quality to them. It was almost as if the leaf could barely contain the life that was now embodied in the plant, and to touch the leaf would cause that life to spring from it.

In early March, a full month ahead of my previous years' schedule, I was told to transplant everything but the tomatoes and green peppers into the garden. I was also told to begin the transplanting at 10 P.M. on a specific day. As instructed by nature, I spent the days prior to that getting the plants ready for the big move by hardening them off (taking the flats outside every day so that the plants could get used to the cold and wind).

On the prescribed evening, I took the flats into the garden and began working. The moon was bright, enabling me to see quite well what I was doing.

The nature spirits began to give me instructions on how to plant without causing the plants to go into shock. I was told that the energy of the plant at night was in the root system, making transplanting at night preferable. During the day, the energy was in the stem and leaves. In human terms, at night the plant was in a state similar to sleep. If I worked quietly, carefully and slowly, the transplanting could be done without disrupting that state. This meant the growth rhythm wouldn't be disturbed.

So there I sat on the mulch in the moonlight with my winter coat, hat and gloves on, transplanting in slow motion. I used a kitchen fork to make a hole just large enough for the root ball, being careful not to stir the soil unnecessarily.

As I worked in this state of slow motion, I felt a penetrating air of peace surround me. I felt as if I were experiencing the LeBoyer Nonviolent Birth Method. I was working in gentle moonlight. No noise. All movement was done with great care. And I could actually sense that the plants were not being disturbed.

I worked in this way until 3 A.M., when finally the job was completed. I left the garden in a deep state of peace and inner quiet that I have been able to duplicate only one other time.

Despite the bitter March cold and wind, the little plants continued to grow at a rapid pace. On the nights when we were due to have a heavy freeze, I would ask the nature spirits to protect the young plants, and the next morning I would go outside to find heavy frost everywhere except on those plants in the garden.

As the planting season continued through April and into May, I got devic information on when to plant specific seeds directly into the garden. I then prepared each row with the help of the nature spirits, planted the seeds, asked that the energies of the vegetable be grounded in the seed and welcomed each new energy into the garden.

The first thing I noticed were the different dynamics and different sensations of each new vegetable energy with which I was connecting. But nothing really surprised me until I connected with the Onion Deva. I had been told that the greatest intensity of energy within the small plants was contained in herbs. That didn't mean much to me until I experienced the Onion Deva that gave me a blast of energy and communication far more intense than anything I had felt up to that point.

In February, while working with nature to plan the garden, I had an insight (no doubt "planted" by my teachers) and wondered if it might be good for the garden's overall balance to include carrots. At the time, my garden soil tended toward clay—Virginia is famous for its brilliant red clay. During the previous years, I had worked on the soil and made it acceptable to most vegetables, but I still couldn't get carrots to grow. Actually, it was more like coaxing carrot seedlings to drill through brick. But this year, I decided it might be good to include carrot energy and not to worry about harvesting the stubby little roots for food. I asked the Overlighting Deva of the Garden if we should include carrots for the sake of the garden's balance and got a "yes."

Nature was so pleased that I had considered something for the sake of balance rather than food demands that they decided to have a little celebration and show their pleasure. When I asked that the carrot energy be grounded into the seed I had just planted, the nature spirits grounded it all right—in every row in the garden! When I opened my eyes and looked into the garden, there before me were three-inch-high carrot plants sticking up everywhere.

I looked at this for a few minutes and then said, "Joke. Right, fellas?! Just fooling around, heh." (I had heard about nature intelligences and their practical jokes.)

Not really wanting a garden of nothing but carrots, I decided I'd call their bluff. So I stretched my hands out and, with a lot of focus, used my hands to "collect" the carrot energy from all the rows into the one row where the seeds were actually planted. Then I said, "No. No. I meant the energy in this row only, thank you."

Instantaneously, the carrot plants in the one row became six inches high—approximately ten minutes after planting the seed—and the carrot plants in the other rows simply fell over and became part of the mulch.

I must say that at this point in the class program, my sense of logic was being severely challenged. Whenever something unusual occurred like the carrot experience, I would take the longest time just to stare at what had happened. I would touch things, I would turn my head away then look back, thinking that the whole thing was an elaborate hallucination and would magically disappear if I looked away from it for a few minutes—but it never disappeared. And that was the point. All these "unusual" events wouldn't disappear. Nor would what I was experiencing fit into any area of my old framework of logic. To put it mildly, these things were not supposed to happen. *They* (all those people who tell you how things are supposed to be) had been telling me that such things did not occur since I was a child. Yet here it was right before me. I had no choice but to accept that what I was perceiving with all my senses was real. And since it didn't fit into my framework of logic, I had to simply "hold" each experience outside that framework. I did not choose to try to force the experience into the framework. I knew that wasn't going to work. So I held them apart from one another and continued on.

As part of my effort to have good, workable soil, I was told to put out the call for earthworms. When it came time to prepare the rows for planting, I discovered an enormous amount of earthworms everywhere I cultivated. That was the good news. The bad news was that it was impossible for me to work the soil without chopping earthworms. We wanted them, we got them, and now I was chopping them. Becoming frustrated and angry at the situation, I stopped cultivating, walked out of the garden and announced out loud, "I'm going to have a fifteen-minute tea break. When I return, I want all of the earthworms that are in this row" (I pointed to the row I had been working in) "to be out of the row. You can be on either side of the row, but not in it."

Then I stomped off for tea, fully expecting nothing whatsoever to come of this. After all, I was only blowing off steam.

I returned, as promised, in fifteen minutes, picked up my hoe and began working in the same row. The earthworms were gone from the entire row. I was as surprised as anyone could possibly have been—and a little spooked by this turn of events.

I finished working the soil and got an insight: If one can "order" earthworms out, one can invite them back in again. So I said, "OK. The coast is clear. I now invite you to come back into the row. I'll give you ten minutes."

I sat down, waited the ten minutes, then went back to the row, picked up several handfuls of soil and found them filled with worms again.

This kind of experience is what I call a "nature setup." Nature sets up a situation that is "designed" to draw a particular response from me. Then nature uses the response as the starting point for the lesson. In this case, I learned something about my own power (and the power we all have) and how nature can interact with that power.

Based on what I was learning about how we can interact directly with nature, I felt my attention being drawn to the moles that had taken over our lawn. Nature directed me to relocate the moles to someplace other than the lawn. Feeling somewhat confident because of the worm experience, I sat down on the grass, got quiet and asked to be connected to the Deva of Moles. I felt a considerable shift but no response. So trusting that the connection was made, I laid out a case about why I thought it would be better for the moles and the lawn if the moles in that area relocated. I explained that I didn't want the moles to leave Perelandra, that I understood they were integral to the life cycle at Perelandra. But would they consider living in the woods or in an open field area about two hundred feet from the house? In either place they could live without being disturbed. Then I suggested that they leave the lawn area at about 9 P.M. Realizing that moles probably couldn't tell time, I changed that to sunset so that they could move to their new areas without being hurt by any of our cats or dogs—who happened to enjoy killing moles. At sunset our animals would be in the house sleeping off dinner.

Still nothing from the Mole Deva.

Assuming my efforts a failure, I returned to the garden. But about a half-hour later, I heard leaves rustling. I looked up and saw a sizable "herd" of moles—at least a hundred in number—scurrying along the woods' edge, heading for the open field area. Both dogs and all three cats ran toward the commotion, and, seeing that there was absolutely nothing I could do to get the five hysterical animals out of the way, I shouted at the moles, "I thought I told you sunset."

Well, it was like dropping a kid in the middle of a four hundred foot high candy mound. The sight of the hundred moles so overloaded the circuits of our animals that they couldn't move. They stood frozen in one spot, making noises and scratching themselves out of frustration, while the moles ran right by them en route to the open field.

In mid-May, I discovered that Peter and Eileen Caddy, two of the co-founders of Findhorn, were on tour in the United States and would be speaking in Virginia at the end of the month. I knew I had to see these two people whose books had so altered my life. Clarence took time off from work, and together we went to their one-day workshop.

I received two important bits of information from the Caddys that day. First, they talked about a three-month program the Findhorn Community was giving that winter called the "Essence of Findhorn." As they spoke about it, I knew I had to go to Findhorn and be a part of that program. Second, I asked Peter what one could do if she has already made a connection with nature and was being run ragged from trying to do everything they wanted. (Since connecting with nature in January, I had made it a point to do everything they suggested as soon as I possibly could. My day was at their mercy, and I was exhausted.) Peter gave me a one sentence answer.

"Remember, *you* are the creator of the garden."

All the way home, I kept saying to myself over and over again, "*I* am the creator of this garden . . . I *am* the creator of the garden . . ." By the time I got home, I believed I was the creator of the garden.

It was never meant for me to be in the role of servant. Rather, I was to eventually take a position of equal partnership with nature. *Equal partnership.* That meant I had to face my own power and responsibility and not see myself as anything less than nature. I was different. Not less.

When I raised this question with nature, I was told that the relationship they seek with humans is an equal, co-creative partnership. I then saw myself as the conductor of an orchestra who was responsible for pulling together all the individual parts into one harmonious whole. That was my role at Perelandra and this was what I was working toward as a co-creative scientist.

Nature told me that I would have to learn to use my power in balance with all that was around me, thus establishing the co-creative partnership. I had to learn that if my power became out of balance with the whole, I would then be working out of manipulation rather than in co-creation. They told me that one of the main reasons Earth was suffering from its present ecological crises was because of man, out of ignorance and arrogance, wielding his power as manipulator of all around him.

I arrived in the garden the next day with a completely different attitude. I came prepared to assume my position of partner—and I came prepared to learn what that meant. I knew I was still a student, but now I had a better concept of what I needed to learn. At nature's urging, I began to address issues that had been bothering me. I first announced that I would no longer be available for little projects at three in the morning. I needed a solid eight hours of sleep and time for personal relaxation, so after leaving the garden at sundown, my "office" would be closed. And I would not be available in the morning until after ten.

To be honest, I half expected nature to "walk out" of the classroom because of my new demands. Instead, the response I received was one of gratitude. Both the devic and nature spirit levels are not human, and they needed me to let them know my needs—my working conditions. They were eager to adjust their contact with me and take into account how I wanted to work. It wasn't that they didn't know me. They were so familiar with me that they geared the information, insights and lessons perfectly to me. But it was important to our working partnership that *I* understood who I was and how I functioned—and to share the information about how I wished to work with them. In short, I had to begin to assume my rightful and proper position in this partnership.

By June, I had developed a consistent daily routine. Each morning I sat on a bench beside the garden with my morning tea. First, I "met" with the devic level by connecting with every deva represented in the garden to find what areas, in some cases what plant, needed attention. I used that information to schedule my day. I would then open myself to the nature spirit level, and we would work together accomplishing the different tasks throughout the day.

All the time I was in the garden, I maintained an inner quiet. With each task, I asked the nature spirits involved how best to do the work. As I worked, I would be given insights about what I was doing and why.

My one disappointment was that I would not be sharing in Findhorn's experience of growing a garden under adverse conditions, thus being able to prove to myself (and to anyone else who saw it) that something different was happening here. Findhorn's gardens were growing in sand. Granted, I had the little situation with the clay, but that wasn't nearly as drastic (or impressive) as sand.

Then in June, the federal government announced that the entire eastern seaboard of the United States was suffering under severe drought conditions, and several of the states (including Virginia) were declared agricultural disaster areas eligible for government assistance. Even with this announcement, I wasn't overly impressed. I was concerned about the plight of the farmers in the area whose fields were turning brown. But the Perelandra garden was completely mulched, and, according to what I had read about mulch gardening, it was protected from drought. What finally caught my attention was a neighbor who called to tell me her mulch garden had burned out. That's when I knew I was working under adverse conditions, and my new acid test was whether or not I would be able to keep this garden thriving using my connections with nature.

Now, I do not for a minute believe that nature decided to wipe out all agriculture in a multi-state area just to verify to me (or anyone who saw my garden) that something special was happening. This is not the kind of thing nature would do. The point is, nature doesn't need to visit catastrophe on many to verify something for one. It has a much better control of form than that. The drought of 1977 was an interesting coincidence that provided some equally interesting observation and insight on my part.

As the summer months pressed on, the drought worsened. The Perelandra garden continued to grow lush and green. My neighbors (the few who visited) began to eye me suspiciously.

About this same time, the cabbage, broccoli, cauliflower and Brussels sprouts plants, now quite large, became heavily infested with cabbage worms, a common problem in our area. In the previous years, I had shifted my counterattack from regular, chemical insecticides to organic methods. But this year, I was told to use neither. A dead bug is a dead bug, whether killed organically or otherwise. I had to consider another solution.

Given my success with the earthworms and moles, nature urged me on by telling me to connect with the Deva of the Cabbage Worm. Following nature's instructions, I announced that I wished to give one plant at the end of each of the four rows to the cabbage worms. Then I requested that the worms remove themselves from all the other plants, except for the four designated plants.

The next morning, all the plants in the four rows were clean of cabbage worms—except for the one plant at the end of each row. What surprised me most was the amount of cabbage worms on the end plants. Each only had the number of worms it could support—the rest that had been in the row (the sheer number of which would have destroyed the designated plants in no time) simply disappeared.

In less than seven days, the other plants had "healed," leaving no holes in their leaves. As a bonus, the designated cabbage plant formed a perfect four-pound head later in the summer.

As the planting progressed during the spring, the overall energy of the garden changed dramatically. Every time a vegetable was added, I could feel a shift in the energy. The cumulative effect was an energy that felt strong and extraordinarily vital.

In early June, in my capacity as "creator of the garden," I led a ceremony at Perelandra. Once again, I had received insight on how to proceed. I declared all of Perelandra a sanctuary for nature intelligence, a sanctuary where it could function in partnership with me in peace, and together we would work toward full balance—whatever this meant. With that, I invited any devas or nature spirits who wished to join us to do so. As soon as I finished my declaration, many different wild-flowers popped up in the woods, and empty flower pots that I had prepared for outdoor flowers were now filled with blooming annuals.

Very soon after this, the intensity of my education was stepped up. I was told by the Overlighting Deva of the Garden that it was important for me, if I wished to continue learning, to gain insight and understanding regarding various dynamics of manifestation. If I were to continue learning about my position as an equal partner, I needed to understand more about what was happening around me and the role I, as a human, played in it. So I continued.

MANIFESTATION: the act, process or an instance of manifesting; to make evident.

MANIFEST: readily perceived by the senses and especially by sight.

I experienced three different dynamics of manifestation.

THE FIRST DYNAMIC: The first one is a common experience among us all. I need something. I state my need. Lo and behold, a big truck rumbles down the road and just as it passes the property, the very thing I need falls out of the truck. Or somebody walks up to me and says, "I think you should have this," and hands me the needed item. Or, we need a new car and only have $100 to spend. We open the Sunday paper to the "For Sale" section, and there is the perfect car and someone needs to get rid of it quickly—for $100.

I needed hay for mulch. The drought had eliminated everyone's first cutting of hay for the season, and the farmers were holding onto every available bale for the next winter. I was told to state precisely what I needed and to picture it exactly. The devas spent time with me on the concept of clear statement and clear imagery. I was told that although this area of manifestation was the one most readily available to us, we generally botch the process by our lack of clarity. We are beginning to catch on to the idea that we have the power to draw our needs to us. But we have not bothered to discipline ourselves enough to use this insight as a consistent tool—our biggest breakdown being clarity. There is a vast difference between stating, "I need some hay" and "I need one ton of grade B mulch hay."

I didn't know the precise tonnage I would need in order to get through the growing season, so I used other means to achieve clarity. First of all, I was told that when considering manifestation, I was always to contact the deva directly involved with the item requested. In this case, it was the Deva of Hay. I was told that I would need hay for two growing seasons—since the drought would cause a hay shortage for the next year as well. Using this information, I asked for enough grade B hay to keep the Perelandra vegetable garden spread six inches deep for two full years.

With that stated, I was instructed to release myself from the process—meaning I was not to be anxious or worry about whether my request had "taken effect." I was to continue my usual daily routine assuming that this particular need would be met. I was to relax and, especially, I was not to use logic to learn where the hay would come from, for that would only place limitations on the manifestation process.

Within a couple of days, a neighbor called and gave us the name and telephone number of a local farmer who had a huge pile of damaged hay that he wanted to get rid of.

The hay lasted us exactly two years.

Clarity of thought, word and visualization were the key points emphasized while I explored the first dynamic of manifestation over and over. When I entered the second dynamic, I found that I also needed these same three key points.

THE SECOND DYNAMIC: In July, I moved into an entirely different dynamic of manifestation. By then, I had an intellectual understanding of how nature worked with energy in order to make something physical to our senses. I understood but I didn't know—I had not experienced—yet.

One afternoon, I was told to verbally request and visualize one cubic foot of a specific manure. (It's called starting with basics!) I might add here that nature did not inform me of what I was about to experience. I was given a series of instructions and I followed them, not knowing where they were leading. By this time, I had developed a high degree of trust for my partner and teacher. My visualization connected me with the deva of this manure who, in turn, pulled together the various energies for the manure. As part of our co-creative partnership, the deva used the specifications in my visualization to determine the amount of manure to be manifested. Then I was told to connect with the nature spirits and follow their direction.

As soon as I connected, I felt myself lift (vibrationally) to a very familiar level—a level I had experienced years before when exploring meditation. There the nature spirits and I waited until, suddenly, I felt a third "presence" enter my awareness. We had been joined by the energy of the manure. With great care, we all three moved "down" in vibration more slowly than I had ever experienced in meditation—or perhaps it was simply more clearly than I had ever experienced. As we moved from one level to the next, I could feel the shift in the manure energy. Eventually, I felt the manure take on a sense of physicalness—I sensed atoms, then molecules, then cells. I sensed form within the nature energy—and eventually, even a slight smell. When I felt it had completed its process, I opened my eyes, and there before me was the cubic foot of manure.

I'm not going to say that I took this casually. For some time, I just stared at the manure, thinking about what had happened. Then I touched it. It was perfectly rotted, finely textured manure—with not much odor, a testament to its well-rotted state. I poked at the pile until I was totally convinced that there was indeed a pile of manure sitting on the ground in front of me. I asked what I was to do with the manure and was told by nature to spread it on the garden where it was needed. (Of course. How silly of me.)

This manifestation process took approximately two hours. It had been "slowed" for my benefit so that I could experience the various sensations. Subsequently, whenever I was invited to join in manifestation, it always took as long as I needed to experience and learn new things about the process, and never was it the same amount of time. Manifestation in its "natural state," shall we say, occurs within that proverbial twinkling of a flea's eye.

After a week's experiences, I was given a variation of this manifestation. This time as the item we were to manifest took on atomic structure, the nature spirits released from the process and let me aid it alone through the final stages into five-senses form. We agreed, on the devic level, to materialize a squash seed, which I then visualized, once again setting off the process. Then, with the nature spirits, I moved to the appropriate level, felt the connection with the seed energy, moved down through the process and, as the seed became atomic, I felt the nature spirits release from my awareness. My initial impulse, which turned out to be correct, was to use my inner focus to "hold" the individual energies together. I could feel that on the atomic level the energies began to mesh together, attracting more to themselves, thus giving the sensation that the package of individual energies was becoming a physical whole. As we moved through the process, that sensation became stronger. I also found that in order for me to properly "hold" the energies together, it was important that my own vibration match their level. In essence, I couldn't assist the energies on the atomic level if my own vibration was geared to one of the other levels.

At the very end of the process, just as the seed was about to become physical, I had to *sharply* intensify my inner focus on the seed energy and once again visualize the actual seed in its physical form. That's when I felt the final sensation of form taking hold within the energy. I opened my eyes and directly before me was the seed.

I was invited to continue working in this particular stage for a couple of weeks. Each day an agreement would be reached between the devic level and myself about a particular need in the garden or around Perelandra—seeds, fertilizers, plants, minerals, tools . . . anything. And then we'd go to work. The quality of focus—the intensity of focus—required from me during the process was greater than I had ever experienced. Sometimes I got sloppy with my focus and everything came to a halt. Sometimes I lost the focus altogether, and the energy package would release, move back to the devic level and disperse into its individual components once again. Sometimes if I wasn't able to pull together the exact amount of intensity needed just prior to the thing becoming physical, I would open my eyes only to find it sitting twenty-five feet or so away from me.

Tools were an interesting lesson. First I had to get over my prejudice against tools actually being part of nature. In this first-year classroom, I didn't yet know how much of the reality around me actually came under nature's domain. But when I began this manifestation work, I found that each tool had a deva, a consciousness. Also, with tools I experienced the de-manifestation process—a reverse action that removed the tool from its physicalness and returned it to its energy state.

THE THIRD DYNAMIC: By the end of July, I was feeling fairly confident about what I was doing. Of course, I wasn't allowed to remain in that state for very long. There was a third dynamic of manifestation yet to come.

This time I was told to open to the devic level. From that level I was "raised" to another level, one that was also very familiar to me. This time I found myself in the Void—a space I had experienced quite a number of times in my earlier meditation work. I was brought out of the Void to the level just "below" it. If the Void is the space where nothing can be distinguished from anything else, not even from myself, yet all that exists is present, then the space just below it is where individuality first takes on its characteristics.

I was told that all the individual energy components that are called together by the deva to form a package come from what I call the Void. In essence, all that is, is created from Oneness. I was also told that on the level just below the Void, I could shift my awareness (through intent) and experience anything else. I could make the shift and share in and experience the consciousness of—for example—a hammer.

This is very difficult to describe in words. It's hard for us to believe that we can actually release from the awareness of our own existence, our own individuality, and share in the reality of something else. But on the level just outside the Void, where individuality is at its point of least delineation, this is quite simple. The key, of course, is having the training and discipline to make this kind of shift in the first place!

With these instructions, my experience with the manifestation process changed. Once there was agreement on what to manifest, I would then shift to that space just below the Void and will myself to share in the consciousness of what was to be manifested. This shift usually took no more that a few seconds. After coming out of that level, I could reflect on what I had learned from the experience, and after considering how I planned to use the item, I could make the decision as to whether or not this particular item would suit the purpose perfectly. Remember, in my role as "creator of the garden" and co-creative partner, whatever I visualized was manifested. Sometimes I made dumb decisions. We'd go through the whole process, and, at the end, I'd find that my original decision had been faulty and what I now had before me was not perfectly suited for the job. This is when demanifestation came in handy. However, by first sharing in the consciousness of the thing, I was able to know beforehand if my decision was correct.

Once I activated the process (after having shifted to the consciousness of the thing and making the decision as to its appropriateness), I opened to the devic level and experienced the various energies being drawn together. I then moved through the levels with the deva, felt the shift to the nature spirits, continued through the process and, at the atomic level, took responsibility for the energy myself until it was form and sitting right in front of me.

My experience with manifestation is not something I take lightly. It is a complex, deep, intense, quiet experience on every level. I never materialized anything without first being instructed to do so. I also got an agreement from the devic level on the precise item to be made physical. From the beginning, I knew that I wasn't experiencing this extraordinary process in order to use it as a tool to "get rich quick" by manifesting indiscriminately. Nor was it meant for me to use as a parlor trick to razzle-dazzle friends. This is a deeply profound experience and not something I would want to cheapen in any way. I have been the recipient of every psychological pressure imaginable, designed to get me to do "just one trick." But I've learned there are three categories of people. One is the group that will hear what I have to say about manifestation, and it will simply hit the right chords and they'll know that manifestation as I have described it is part of reality. The second group are the fence-sitters. They won't make a decision one way or the other unless they see just one more piece of evidence . . . and one more piece . . . and one more piece. . . . The third group are the confirmed skeptics. They are particularly adept at trying to pressure me. If I do it just one time for them, they'll believe, etc., etc.

If I manifested an elephant, the first group would consider my action unnecessary, even frivolous and disrespectful. The second group would say, "That's fine. But let's see you manifest a sherman tank." The third group, after goading me into action, would then accuse me of dabbling in Las Vegas magic and brand me a charlatan. I'd end up with a confused elephant and three groups of dissatisfied people glaring at me.

I didn't experience manifestation for this. In order for me to continue my work with nature on a deeper level, I had to know, down to my very core, what it meant for something to become physical to our five senses—that the principle of creation is not just reserved for humans. It is a process shared by everything. If I were to truly understand the foundations of co-creative science, I'd have to learn to respect all life, all things around me in a new way. This meant I had to experience the levels of creation and manifestation.

Several people have suggested that I not share with others my experiences with manifestation. They fear that someone will take my information and use their power to force something to materialize. In essence, they might use their power to manipulate. And manipulation is exactly the thing we need to get away from. It's the thing nature has to deal with constantly when dealing with humans. We know very well how to use our power to manipulate the reality around us to conform to our personal whims. But I feel we can no longer shy away from the universal laws of manifestation. We need to understand this aspect of our reality if we are to become equal partners with all on Earth.

Since my third year in nature's classroom, I have not participated in the kind of manifestation processes that I have described in the second and third dynamics in this book. Once the lessons were over, they were over. I haven't been tempted to "practice" this type of manifestation because of the deep feelings about the experiences that I have and the simple fact that the first dynamic I described is all one needs to understand and practice for everyday life. Be clear about what is needed, state that need clearly, and then release from the process, knowing that what you have defined and described is on its way. The catch seems to be this release issue. We like to determine how we wish to obtain something. (This is another example of how we try to do nature's job.) We'll take it if it's left by a stranger on the front porch but not by a neighbor on the back porch. Or, we want it only if it is free. We don't want to consider the opportunity of earning the money that will enable us to actually purchase the thing. This simple manifestation, which is nothing more than i/e balance in action, works well when it is used correctly and we remain flexible to all the different options that might come our way for achieving our stated goals. And, to be honest, it is actually a lot easier to pull off than dynamics two and three. Once you felt the exhaustion from all the focus that is required in these two dynamics, you'd be happy to accept the more simple route of dynamic one. It would feel like a vacation to you.

My summer of my first-year classroom was not yet over.

One day nature told me to hold a yellow squash in my hands. I was told to just watch it sitting in my hands. I'd say I had been looking at it for about five minutes when, right before my eyes, the yellow squash turned into a green cucumber that was slightly larger in size than the squash had been. The switch took less than fifteen seconds. And it was gradual, so I knew that someone had not sneaked up on me and switched the squash with a cucumber while I blinked. I saw the squash actually change into a cucumber. Now, this was a new affront to my already sorely tested logic. Somewhere along the line I had been taught that if you pick up a squash and hold it in your hands, chances were it would remain a squash. It was one of those assumptions I had grown to trust. Here nature was showing me that this wasn't necessarily the case. Form could change. And nature could change the form of anything it wanted—at any time.

I have to tell you, holding a squash that turns into a cucumber right before your eyes is a dumbfounding experience. Particularly if you haven't been forewarned. I just stared at the thing for a good half hour, trying to get my wits about me. As I have said, I deal with events like this by saying, "Hold on. Nobody move. Let me get this." Then I just stare and touch and sniff until I am completely convinced that what I am presently seeing, feeling and smelling is what I think it is. I did this a lot that first summer. I don't want you to think

I moved through these kinds of experiences without batting an eye. While looking at this cucumber, I even accused nature of not playing by the rules. Of course, that was the point. Whose rules were we talking about here? Just as I was getting used to the cucumber, they changed it back to the yellow squash. (I never ate that squash. I just wasn't sure if the thing that ended up on my plate would be the thing I cooked. I mean, what if I started out—in good faith—steaming the squash, and ended up with a plate of steamed watermelon or turnips. Actually, I was a little nervous about everything I harvested from the garden that year!)

Just as our sweet corn crop began to tassel, it was attacked—ravaged is more to the point—by Japanese beetles. They ate the pollen and demolished the silk. Now, the normal process with corn is that the pollen falls from the tassel onto the silk, thus pollinating the silk. It's the pollination of the silk that causes each kernel of the ear to fill out. Without pollen and silk, one ends up with an ear of corn with no kernels. This summer, if I wanted to salvage any corn, I had to deal with the Japanese beetles.

Reading my concern, nature suggested I contact the Deva of the Japanese Beetle. Much to my astonishment, I touched into an energy that I can only describe as that of a battered child. It was an energy of defeat, of being beaten into submission. Yet it still had mixed in with it anger and a strong desire to fight for its life.

I was told by the deva that what I was experiencing was not devic but from the consciousness of the Japanese beetle itself. I needed this experience in order to understand what our relationship with the beetle had already done to it before I made any requests on the devic level about removing it. You see, the Japanese beetle is not indigenous to the United States. It was introduced to our country by one person who brought in several beetles to be part of his insect collection but accidentally released them. They do not have enough natural predators here, and they have multiplied into a serious problem for our agricultural industry. Consequently, for the past fifty years or so, we have waged a war against the beetle. What I touched into was the result of that war.

Under the circumstances, I felt I had no right to ask anything of the beetle. So I simply asked that the beetle recognize Perelandra as a sanctuary and invited it to join us so that it could begin to heal—whatever that meant. I stated that we would not damage or destroy the beetles and would make every effort to enhance its healing process. To seal the bargain, so to speak, I stated that we would leave unmowed a specific area of tall grass that was a favorite of the beetle.

I then addressed the issue of the corn. Still hoping to salvage some of it, I decided I would try to raise the vibration of the individual stalks—perhaps the ears would fill out in spite of the Japanese beetle. And, with this, I stumbled into another nature setup. I spent three days putting my hands on each stalk and LOVING it. At the end of three days, nature had had enough of this nonsense and I was told to leave the corn patch and not return "until further notified."

Nature intelligence does not respond to "gooey, sentimental love." Nature's love is a love of action and purpose, and it is that kind of active love it desires from us. (Once while giving a workshop, I was asked to accompany several of the leaders of this particular community to a bush. It was a large bush, and it didn't take a horticulturist to see that it was dying. It seems they had recently transplanted the bush, and, as part of their transplanting process, several members in the community would form a circle around it each evening, join hands and send the bush love . . . LOVE. The bush had the nerve to start to die on them anyway. I was asked what they should do. I walked up to the bush, looked at the soil around it, checked the leaves, then turned around and said, "Try watering it." That's love in action. Not to be confused with loveless action. Love in action is appropriate action done in a caring spirit.)

I stayed away from the corn patch for three weeks, until one morning I was told to return. I found that every ear of corn had filled out—but not fully. Only half filled out. The devic pattern of this corn had shifted, making it possible for the ears to mature without using the natural tassel/pollinated silk process. I was told that half the ear had matured because this planting of corn was to be fed to the birds at Perelandra for the winter, and only the amount that was needed matured. A later planting standing right next to this corn, and not yet damaged by the beetle, would be for our use exclusively and would be allowed to fully mature in the natural process.

A month later, the second planting matured untouched.

In the years since making the agreement with the Japanese beetle, I notice that they have increasingly become more calm and fewer in number. For several years, they damaged only the roses. Still, I didn't disturb them. It wasn't easy, since my natural impulse was to whack them off the rose bushes. But after some mental adjustments on my part, I could actually invite them to enjoy the roses. Now they do not "flock" to the roses, but I'll still see a manageable number on the bushes from time to time. Because of the shifts and changes on the part of the beetles and the gardener, I've found that I have not had reason to request anything special from them. Their presence here feels in balance.

Starting in mid-August that summer, my days became quite difficult to manage. I received word from Findhorn that I had been accepted into the Essence of Findhorn program. I was to report to Findhorn the first week of November. That gave me a little over two months to get the food in for the winter, prepare for my trip to Scotland and close down the garden.

With these pressures, I changed my attitude toward the way I approached the garden. I no longer had time for leisurely morning teas, and I certainly didn't have time to do everything in the garden that was being suggested. So I tended to enter my morning devic meetings much like a drill sergeant. "OK. What needs to be done?" (Listen.) "Fine. I'll do that, that and that, but the other stuff will have to wait."

Soon after this, I arrived one morning to find that the row of Brussels sprouts plants—that had grown to stand a perfect three feet tall—had been attacked by a horde of bugs, leaving the leaves badly damaged and the plants weak.

I couldn't believe what I was seeing. I connected with the Deva of the Brussels Sprout to find out what was going on.

When you look at the garden now, you see a half-empty glass. You focus on the negative. You deal in only the work to be done. You no longer see the beauty and what is being accomplished here. Your attitude has unbalanced the energy of the garden, leaving it vulnerable to being overpowered and destroyed by insects. Since you have altered the balance, it is important for you to reestablish the balance. You must understand the power contained in thoughts and attitudes and the integral part they play in the balance of the whole.

I needed to return to the garden, but more importantly, I needed to recapture the attitude that I had had throughout the summer. It wasn't easy. I found it quite difficult to drop all else and refocus exclusively on the garden.

It took me three days to rebalance the garden. Mostly, I concentrated on seeing the garden in terms of its accomplishments and beauty—and how much I was learning. At the end of the three days, the bugs had vanished from the Brussels sprouts plants, and the plants had started a healing process.

Now the key to maintaining the garden's balance was attitude. It wasn't the amount of work that had thrown the energy off, it was the attitude with which I was working: Pressed. Concerned. Worried. Anxious about the trip. When I finally left to spend more time with my other responsibilities, I made it a point to move in and out of the garden in a clear, settled, quiet state of mind. With this, the garden balance held.

I felt from nature that it was important to wait until after the first heavy frost and not rush the job of "putting the garden to bed"—that is, preparing the garden for winter. I waited and waited for that frost, and for awhile it looked as if I would have to set off for Findhorn, leaving this last job for Clarence.

Finally the frost hit. I moved into the garden to do the last process, thus completing the season's cycle.

What I had assumed would take one day actually took seven full days. It was a most extraordinary experience, very similar to the nonviolent birth experience I felt when first planting that early spring night. Only this time, it was nonviolent death. I spent seven days touching into each energy that had become part of the garden. I thanked it for its presence, then released it from the garden. I found that even if the form of the plant was dead, the energy, the consciousness of the plant, had remained a part of the whole energy of the garden. As I released it—either by removing the plant or touching into the energy and simply requesting that it release—I felt it leave my own awareness. The nature intelligence of that vegetable then released from the garden. Everything had to be done gently and slowly, respecting the fact that this growing cycle was over, and we were going into a period of rest and peace. The atmosphere around me was calm—very calm. Every move I made was slow but deliberate and precise—it was clarity in motion. All the time, I stayed in contact with the specific consciousness with which I was working.

It's difficult to communicate this experience because of its depth, its mixture of peace, gentleness and love, and because it was happening on different levels simultaneously, both inside me and outside me. In retrospect . . . it had to be the deepest time.

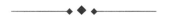

This was my first year in a co-creative science classroom. From that garden, I started learning about the universal laws of nature and how they apply to the form around me. I also started learning about partnership, teamwork, leadership and peer relationships. And as much as I learned about universal laws, nature and these other things, I learned about my-self—my power, equality, balance, health, heart and soul.

As you can see, the class setup was simple. Nature would give me something specific to do. I would then do it, observe the results, then sometimes receive more instructions about what to do next. Again I'd do what I was told and observe the results. Often, I got the understanding of what nature was try-ing to teach me simply through the conclusions I could draw from doing and observing. The act itself became the explana-tion. At other times, I would act, observe and still be blank regarding what I was seeing. That's when nature would some-times "step in" and give me the additional insight I needed for understanding.

And then there were those times when I would act, ob-serve, stare blankly and *not* receive any insight. I would close the day not understanding anything I did. That's when I'd scratch my head a lot. I'd come back the next day, open to na-ture and start the whole process over again. I may end up with a string of days where I had absolutely no understanding about what I was doing or observing. But I'd keep plugging along. Eventually, I'd observe something I had just done and this would be the piece I needed to pull that day and all the previous blank days together into one large, comprehensible package. I'd finally get it.

Nature taught me that life is a learning process that doesn't necessarily include comprehension at given points along the way, and that one must proceed in this process in faith and with patience. I experienced from nature a complete reversal of just about everything I thought I knew, including many things I took for granted. In hindsight I realize that nature was carefully dismantling my previous sense of logic and replacing it with a completely different and more expanded logic. And nature was doing this by giving me the actual experiences rather than "lectures" about such experiences.

A point about talking to others about these experiences: I talked to Clarence about what was happening in the early part of the season—the late winter, early spring months. To my amazement, he didn't show any evidence that he thought I was mentally disturbed. But as the lessons intensified, I became more quiet and I stopped sharing with him. I just needed to keep it to myself. He continued to support me by not questioning what I was doing and not getting in my way. It was the best kind of support I could have. To this day, I remain quiet about the things I am learning until I feel it's time to "go public" with the information.

When I went to Findhorn, I had thought it was so that I could continue learning about how to work with nature. But I quickly discovered that my own garden experiences at Perelandra were all the lessons I needed and that Findhorn would not be a part of this education. Instead, Findhorn gave me an opportunity to see that I could share my experiences in a more public way, if I wanted. What was happening to me at Perelandra was of interest to others, and they could learn from what I could talk about. I tucked that information into "my back pocket" and returned to Perelandra and my second year in nature's class.

The second year, of course, was totally different from the first. I went through the same procedure with nature to get the garden to the point where everything was planted. Then nature told me not to do anything else for the garden for the rest of the season, except harvest. Each day I was to walk down all the rows and observe. They didn't say what to observe, just to do it. I thought nature was crazy, quite frankly. (It's OK to think these things. Nature doesn't take it personally.) Each day during the summer weeks, I'd stroll along the rows in the garden. To be honest, the garden looked like hell. Weeds were growing everywhere. Some plants were overrun with insects. And some plants could not have looked happier. I had no idea what was going on. When I asked for a hint from nature, they'd say, "You'll see." Throughout the summer, we had a number of visitors from Findhorn who stopped by to see the "famous" Perelandra garden. They'd look at this mess and say things like, "Gee, I know a fellow who is a really fine gardener. Maybe you'd like to talk to him. I'll give you his phone number." Instead of taking my cue from nature and replying that this is what nature wanted me to do this year, and that I trusted that it would eventually make sense to me, I told them what I *thought* was going on. Of course, I was completely off base.

Unlike the previous year, I was pretty happy to put this garden to bed.

In 1979, my third year, the garden was back to having order. Nature was giving me all kinds of different information about what needed to be planted where and how to tend to everything throughout the season. Just after the garden was planted, it dawned on me what the previous year had been all about. It was a fact-finding year. Nature had me plant the garden, then back away so that it (nature) and I could observe what happens to that garden's balance when left on its own within a specific environment. While nature was doing an environmental impact study, I was watching the results of the study playing out in the garden. So now, as I moved into this new garden, I understood why nature was making so many changes and what was behind the changes.

In the spring of that year, I intuitively sensed that I needed to dedicate myself to taking the next step with nature. I didn't know what the next step was, but I knew I was not supposed to ask. I was simply supposed to decide if I wanted to go on, then announce my decision. I thought it over a bit. I didn't see any reason to back away from this adventure. So, one afternoon I announced that I wanted to go on to the next step. It was as simple as that.

In midsummer, I was told to move the garden from its present location beside the house to an open-field area four hundred feet away. It was to be done by the next gardening season. Well. Moving a garden is a chore. I didn't know how I was going to break the news to Clarence (I'd need his help), so I didn't say anything for several weeks. Then one day, as Clarence and I were returning from a walk, he looked right at the "proposed" new site and said, "You know, that's a much better location for the garden." Sensing an advantageous moment, I told him about the move. He said that in the fall we could get one of the local farmers to come plow the field for the new garden.

"The next step" moved me from a private, family-oriented gardening student seeking to work in partnership with nature to a co-creative nature research student using a garden as her laboratory. Much of my efforts in 1980 (the fourth year class) were centered around getting the new garden in place and settled. It was three times larger than the old one and consisted of eighteen concentric circles—the last of which was one hundred feet in diameter. Clarence built a small shed/office for me, and I worked every weekday from the time he left Perelandra in late morning until after sundown.

The fifth year, 1981, nature and I began developing the many processes that I eventually wrote about in the *Perelandra Garden Workbook*. Nature instructed me on how to set up a coning—an interlevel energy vortex that contains balance between the involution and evolution dynamics—and I began to have all my nature sessions while in conings.* I also began fine-tuning my ability to translate longer tracts of information from nature.

In my sixth year, I received two instructions from nature: (1) Set up an office in the house; (2) Take an R&R for six to nine months. I was still to plant the garden that year, but the time I needed for the garden classroom was dramatically reduced so that I could take advantage of the R&R. Setting up the office provided an interesting surprise. I had not realized how many notes, charts and pages of session information I had collected over the past five years in this class until I set up that first office and began to centralize all the information into files.

---

* If you wish to know more about setting up and working in a coning, see the following publications: the two *Perelandra Garden Workbooks*, *MAP* and the *Perelandra Microbial Balancing Program Manual*.

My seventh year was a relatively quiet year in the garden. Nature and I focused on the continuing business of developing the co-creative processes for working in a garden that grows in soil or in one that is soil-less. This summer, I felt my relationship with my partner changing. Although I knew there would always be something for me to learn from nature, I could feel that I was no longer nature's student. I was now nature's partner in co-creative science. There was a difference in the give and take that occurred between us. I was not posturing myself as the student. And I could feel that nature was not "posturing" itself as my classroom teacher. I felt myself automatically step into my role as the partner who provides the direction, definition and purpose for the work we do together. I was able to *clearly* see the many changes I had gone through because of my classroom work with nature.

1. I had changed my framework of logic dramatically. I now saw reality and how it works with new eyes—from nature's perspective.

2. I had a good sense of the extraordinary depth of nature's knowledge about reality.

3. I had over six years of positive (and often amazing) results from the many lessons and processes that I had experienced with nature. This wasn't happening in my head. I had observed all the results in the garden.

4. I now knew how to address a problem and set up research with nature for resolving the problem in a balanced and environmentally sound way.

5. I had deep confidence about moving through each process as nature was instructing me to move despite my not having a clue about what I was doing.

6. I knew how to troubleshoot a mistake or misunderstanding and work with nature to correct the situation. This was a critical element that I had to learn for our partnership.

7. I knew that in order to really understand something, I needed to experience it from nature's perspective—to work with it, observe and listen. This new way of looking at reality is so different, we could not accurately understand something if nature simply gave us a lecture about it. We wouldn't know how to hear what was being said. Our ability to perceive must change to match nature's different knowledge and understanding before we can understand. Otherwise, we wouldn't have the necessary tools in place and we would superimpose our old understanding onto the words and insights that nature gives us.

8. I had in place an efficient and excellent working structure and laboratory for doing research with nature. We had developed many bridges or tools of communication: kinesiology, charts for efficiently transferring information, insight, intuition, gut instinct, visual insight, sudden thoughts from out of nowhere. . . . And I was developing my written translation skills that resulted in understanding nature in deeper ways. Also, I now had a strong ability to ignore outside "advice" from others as to how scientific research "should be done." I knew I had the best research laboratory around.

But I had one ongoing debate that still raged on. By 1980, I understood that I was moving in a direction with nature that was "professional oriented" and not private. I was not going through this class just so I could be a well-informed nature lover. I saw that something important was happening. But I didn't know how it would fit into the larger societal picture. As I saw it, society wasn't going to accept this into its picture at all. It was too different—too nuts. I kept thinking I should take time out to "get some recognized credentials" in chemistry, botany, biology—at least something from one of the soil sciences. Surely this would make me a "better educated" individual for nature to work with, plus give me the recognition needed in the larger society. I struggled with this debate for years. Nature kept telling me that I didn't need these credentials, that they were non-issues. I'd hear this, settle down a bit, and then something would come to my attention and the old debate would rise again. It made me feel irresponsible as a developing scientist. I didn't settle the debate until 1989, when I met a scientist who had many of those credentials and who said—after looking hard at my research and setup, and studying my papers and notes for months—that I would not benefit at all from stopping what I was doing with nature and going into a conventional study program. It would not be helpful to my research. In short, a university program could give me no useful information and I would only have to forget everything I learned in order to continue my research with nature. He suggested that I already had the best teacher and best partner a scientist could ever want. His input helped me to understand nature's advice in this matter, and I put the debate to rest.

———————◆ ◆ ◆———————

SETTING UP A CO-CREATIVE
SCIENCE CLASS WITH NATURE

Everyone's class will be different. This is the first thing you will have to address if you enter nature's science class. Although nature teaches all of us the same principles and universal laws, how it teaches them will be somewhat different because nature tailors the information and lessons to the individual and how much he can handle, observe and hear at any given time. I suggest that you enter this class alone and not try to set up something for several students at one time. In this situation, nature will take into consideration the group as a whole and you will lose the advantage of the personal attention that nature can give. This means that the lessons and insights won't be moving along according to your personal timing and rhythm because the group dynamic will always be a factor. However, this doesn't mean that a group of you can't set up individual classrooms with nature and then meet periodically to discuss what is happening in your respective classes. Although this could be supportive and helpful, you each must keep in mind at all times that the classes will be presented differently, and the range and scope of subject matter will depend on what is needed for the individual. In short, you would be doing more harm than good if you got into a competition with one another about who you felt was moving along more quickly, who was having the "neat" experiences and who was the teacher's "favorite."

About my classes: It would be nuts to expect nature to give you your classes as it gave me mine. I admit I had some extraordinary experiences, and I'm sure many others would like to have these experiences as well. But keep in mind that I had no books to give me any kind of foundation in this education. This is not your situation. And the path that we were moving down was new not just to me, but to nature also. In a real sense, my education had to "come out of the blue." I think it is fair to say that things needed to be presented in a "big way" just so I could get it. We were developing the bridge for communicating as we went along and we weren't sure what was going to work in each situation. Now you have the advantage of moving down this path and benefiting from the material we have published as well as from my experiences. I feel certain that your education will move even more efficiently and smoothly. After all, it took me seven years to complete this classroom education, and nature is now estimating that it will take you about four years. Try your best not to get into a competition with my experience and keep your focus on what is unique and amazing about your own experiences with nature. I have presented my experiences in order to give you an idea of the scope that is involved, not so you can aim to duplicate them. If you try, you will only end up frustrated and disappointed—and your teacher will give you an F for class participation.

The time that you spend in class depends on you. I made this a priority in my life and spent hours every day focused on the classroom itself or thinking about what I was learning while away from the classroom. But I was in a situation where I could devote this kind of time. I didn't have to work outside Perelandra and I didn't have children to care for. You must take your own variables into consideration. If you are choosing to train as a co-creative scientist, you cannot be making this move on a lark. You wouldn't just wake up one morning and announce, "By gosh, I think I'll study to be a brain surgeon today." It is assumed that you are as serious about this commitment as you would be about any other professional commitment. So, think about your personal responsibilities. Then consider how you would have to adjust your schedule in order to pursue an education from a university for a comparable "normal" professional change. Would you be willing to make those changes in your daily schedule to accommodate such a professional change? If not, consider that at this point in your life, you do not have the time to take on the education required for a co-creative scientist. Return to the question later on in your life when your circumstances have changed. In short, taking on the rigors of a co-creative science education should not be viewed as a hobby just because its classroom is not in a formalized educational structure such as a university and you will not be required to take exams or write papers. If you are willing and able to make changes in your schedule, apply the time you would have committed to achieving the education for a "normal" professional change to the co-creative science classroom. For example, if you could have taken one or two courses three evenings a week for four or five years, go ahead and apply this same amount of time to the co-creative classroom and rearrange your life to accommodate that commitment.

The primary communication bridge that you will be using is kinesiology, the muscle-testing technique that I have already mentioned. I suggest that you learn to use kinesiology before setting up a classroom with nature. That way you will be able to communicate with nature right away. It doesn't take long to learn and you don't need to become an expert before entering the class. You only need to be able to discern a clear "yes" and "no" using the testing technique. (Remember, the steps for learning kinesiology are in the appendix.)

This is how nature uses the kinesiology bridge with us. We ask nature a simple question that requires a "yes" or "no" answer. Nature then projects that "yes" or "no" to us, which then registers as a positive or negative in our body's electrical system. This is easy for nature to do because it is working with intelligence and using the natural dynamic as described in Chapter 2: flow. Nature *flows* its "yes" or "no" response to us. The flow impacts our electrical systems, which respond by registering the "yes" or "no." Thus nature utilizes a process that is natural to all of us. We use the kinesiology testing technique to "read" nature's answer from our electrical system. It is a simple technique, it is efficient, and it is effective. I recommend that this technique be learned and used when working with nature, especially in the beginning. After a year or two, you will notice a sharpening of your intuition and your ability to pick up visual and thought insight. The foundation for these developments lies with learning and using kinesiology well. As you improve your kinesiology testing, you will experience an extensive internal "housecleaning" and reorganization that will result in a sharpening of these other tools. It is important that you not deliberately aim to fine-tune the other tools. Just concentrate on learning to use kinesiology well. Although it does not take you long to learn how to discern a positive and negative response with the testing, it does take about a year to learn how to use the technique well for a wide range of situations. You'll have plenty of situations to practice your testing on in the classroom.

Getting Started in the Classroom

This is the easy part. I am assuming that you have assessed your situation, made your commitment and learned how to discern a simple "yes" and "no" using kinesiology, and that you are now ready to initiate the co-creative classroom with nature. Here's what to do:

1. VERBALLY STATE YOUR INTENTION TO NATURE. I recommend that you state this out loud. Nature doesn't need to hear it out loud. As an intelligence, it doesn't have ears. However, I have found that when we say something aloud instead of just keeping it in our heads, we are clearer and we can listen to what we are saying. When I'm working with nature, I often speak out loud just for the sake of clarity, and sometimes it helps me maintain focus.

Your statement does not have to be elaborate. In fact, the simpler the better. *Focus your attention on nature and its intelligence* (just think about it) and say something like:

"I would like to open a co-creative science classroom with myself as the student and nature intelligence as my teacher. My intent is to be educated and trained as a co-creative scientist. I am ready to learn."

Then I recommend that you make a four- to six-month time commitment with nature. Simply state how many hours a week and on what days and at what times you plan to focus with nature in the classroom during this period. This commitment is important not just for you, but for nature as well. It sets up the physical time and rhythm you plan to be present for in the classroom. This way, nature will be able to "plan" the class work according to your rhythm. When the first period is over, assess your time commitment and schedule the next four to six months. Keep this going until the class is completed—in about four or five years.

2. SELECT YOUR CLASSROOM. Of course, I recommend a garden, if at all possible. It is an excellent environment for learning about the laws of nature. It has a built-in annual cycle that is conducive to this class's rhythms. It provides quick feedback when you are working in it—either the plant you are working on improves or it croaks. There is nothing ethereal and uncertain about a garden. It also provides a structure for constant movement, and nature teaches us well when we are moving along in an activity. On top of all of this, you can eat things from it—if it is a vegetable garden. Another point: You do not need to know how to garden in order to select a garden as your classroom. In fact, the less you know, the less you will have to overcome or forget. The *Perelandra Garden Workbook* and the *Perelandra Garden Workbook II* give you the complete guidelines for working with nature in a garden.

If you hate the idea of gardening or you don't have any place to put in a garden, choose another classroom. It will have to be something that provides a structure for action: athletic training, home management, automotive mechanics, pond management, landscaping, greenhouse management, furniture making. . . . Pick something that you can do alone, and remember that whatever you choose will become a classroom and you will need to hand over all the activity, timing and rhythms to your teacher. So, don't choose something you are not willing to release control of and don't pick something that is life-threatening either to yourself or anyone else. Your classroom has to remain personal for the amount of time you and nature are using it, so I suggest you not choose something that will drive your "significant other" crazy because you have usurped some shared space as your own. You will still be using the two *Perelandra Garden Workbooks* as your guidelines for establishing the working class relationship with nature no matter what you choose, but you will have to "translate" the *Workbooks* as you go along to apply the language relating to gardening to your classroom. We include information with the *Workbooks* on how to do this.

3. BEGIN READING AND STUDYING THE MATERIAL THAT IS PUBLISHED BY PERELANDRA. You will need to begin with the two *Perelandra Garden Workbooks*. These are your first texts and nature will begin working with you as you apply this material to your chosen classroom. There is quite a bit of Perelandra material for you to work with, but you do not need everything on hand at one time. Request a list of publications from Perelandra (the address and phone numbers for requesting our catalog are in the back of this book), and go through the list with your teacher. Ask nature what material you should get after the *Workbooks* and kinesiology test the list. (How to do this is explained in the *Workbooks*.) Whatever tests positive is what nature recommends you work with next.

NOTE: If you have already read and worked with the two *Workbooks* and now wish to open a co-creative science classroom, you will still need to choose a classroom and work with the two books within that class situation. Even if you have been applying these books successfully to your garden for years and wish to use that garden as your classroom, remember that the garden ceases to be a regular garden once the classroom is initiated. It is now a classroom and its timing and rhythms will change. In short, don't assume that what you have experienced in the garden with nature previously will be what you will experience with it in the classroom. You now have a different environment and situation with nature and you will be starting your work fresh.

You have now entered your co-creative science classroom and begun your education with nature. From this point, it's between you and nature. However, if you somehow "paint yourself in a corner" and can't figure out how to work with nature to get out of it, you can call the Perelandra Question Hot Line for suggestions about what to do. The phone number and the times that this line is open are published in the Perelandra Catalog. We will be glad to get you up and moving again with nature in your classroom.

IMPORTANT: Keep *good* notes. Keep a log of what you do each day in class and what you observe. Also include any insights or questions you have about what you are doing. And make sure you record anything you learn, including insights and information you get from nature. These notes organize you and your thoughts as you move through the class. You will want to refer to them often. They will help you see your progress over the years and they will serve as the foundation of information that you will refer to once you begin functioning as a co-creative scientist. There are two keys to keep in mind for these notes: (1) Be complete. Keep a full record of everything. (2) Be organized. Your notes will not be useful if they are scribbled on bits of paper and dumped into a box.

How to Determine When You Have Completed
Your Co-Creative Science Class

In Chapter 3, I listed the twelve skills a co-creative scientist needs and, in this chapter, I listed eight changes I could clearly recognize at the end of my seven years in the class. These two lists provide excellent guidelines for what one needs in order to function with nature as a co-creative scientist. My experience with the information on the two lists is that when it was time to "leave the classroom," there was no question in my mind about the changes I had gone through and what I now understood. I was confident in these matters—and it was a quiet, deep confidence. It wasn't a confidence of the ego, rather, it was of the mind and heart.

The twelfth skill (in Chapter 3) states that the co-creative scientist "must have a balanced sense of ego and self-worth, and a personal commitment to honesty and overall integrity." We have no recognizable "graduation" ceremonies in co-creative science—yet. A student must intend to complete the course, and possess the honesty, integrity and dedication to stay in the class until the course is completed. "Graduation" occurs between nature and the individual student. In fact, when the class work is completed, nature automatically shifts from a teacher/student relationship to a peer partnership in co-creative science. For the student, that shift, although felt from within, is clear and undeniable, and the new work that occurs between them changes accordingly. The criteria for the shift is our understanding of our role with nature and our ability to function in that role within the partnership in science.

Of course, we in society will be able to tell if the person really graduated or if he decided it was time for graduation whether he was ready or not by the quality of the work he does as a co-creative scientist. If his processes don't work, create confusion or cause more problems than they solve, he never finished the course with nature. This is someone who went to a lot of trouble to look like a co-creative scientist, but then took over control of the class and partnership and relegated nature to "the back seat."

Even if in the future universities offer co-creative science as a course from which a student may graduate, the real graduation will still not be on a stage with odd-looking caps and gowns and lots of beaming relatives. The real graduation will be between nature and the student. This is a science that is taught by nature. It is a working partnership that is formed between nature and the student. A university curriculum will never replace this in co-creative science.

Do I think that co-creative science can be offered in universities? Yes. There are published texts to be read and many discussions to be had. However, a co-creative *scientist's* primary education can only be given by nature. It won't take a change in procedure for a university to acknowledge co-creative science as a valuable part of everyone's education. But the university professors who wish to assist in educating students as co-creative scientists will have to learn how to work with those students in conjunction with nature. They will need to help the students set up their individual nature classrooms and support them through their education process with nature. To do this, the professor himself will need to gain the skills and insights from his own classroom work with nature. I guarantee that if university professors can learn to work in conjunction with nature's classes, it will make for much more interesting and relevant science courses.

5

Practical Co-Creative Science for the Non-Scientist Facing Everyday Problems

T HE CO-CREATIVE SCIENTIST WORKS with nature to develop grand-scale solutions for current problems and issues. But he can apply these solutions himself only so far. He
relies on the co-creative non-scientists to educate themselves,
to learn to use the different solutions the scientist has worked
out with nature and then apply those solutions to the specific
problem situations as they impact the non-scientists' immediate world and everyday life. As a result, a vibrant and vital
relationship develops between the co-creative scientist and the
non-scientists. In co-creative science, there are no magic pills
that can be administered to everyone for eliminating a single
global problem. Instead, co-creative science recognizes the individual circumstances within all life, and its solutions have
built into them a respect and consideration for this individuality. A scientist working with nature may develop a process or

program that can be used globally for specific problems, such as the Perelandra Microbial Balancing Program that addresses microbial problems in our health and environment. But when a co-creative program such as this is used by individuals for their microbial problems, the results of the testing of each of the steps in the program vary with each person and each situation. Every person's and every environment's needs for having balance restored are different. Yet the final overall impact of a co-creative program such as the Perelandra Microbial Balancing Program is the same globally—balance in our health and environment. In short, a co-creative solution addresses the uniqueness within all environments, all gardens.

A co-creative scientist may work on specific projects in which the solution results in a change of public policy that in turn improves the lives of the non-scientists and their environment, thus not requiring the immediate participation of the non-scientist in order to achieve wholesale change and improvement. In these cases, we have improvement "by default." Society does not have to actively participate in order to receive the benefits of a scientific solution. It only needs to accept those benefits. But, because of co-creative science's unique approach to problems, most of its solutions do require societal participation in order to achieve wholesale change and improvement, thus creating that special relationship between the co-creative scientist and the individual members of society. In co-creative science, the non-scientists' participation is critical to this science's success. They are the implementors. They are the ones who affect broad-scale change. The scientist working with nature develops the guidelines and steps for change, but without the participation of the non-scientists the promise and potential of those solutions do not become actualized until the non-scientists integrate them into their lives and implement them into everyday situations.

The non-scientist does not have to spend years of his life studying and working with nature. He only needs a solid belief in the direction and goals of co-creative science, a willingness to read and learn, and the ability to follow the simple steps that are laid out in the different processes and programs. Another way of saying this is that the non-scientist doesn't develop solutions, he implements them after they have been developed. As a result, he improves the health and well-being of himself and those around him and of his environment. As an individual using the co-creative solutions, he has a tremendously positive impact on his immediate world. Collectively, non-scientists intensify their impact—they can change the larger world.

It is important that non-scientists understand their role and the important part they play in co-creative science. It is also important that they understand the role of the co-creative scientist and his work with nature. The solutions are carefully developed and tested by these two partners in science and meet the high standards of co-creative science. It is irresponsible and counterproductive for non-scientists to attempt to function in the role of the scientist and arbitrarily change the processes beyond the guidelines set by nature and the scientist in order to satisfy his (the non-scientist's) personal tastes and whims. The role of the non-scientist in co-creative science is important, but it does not include any of the responsibilities of the co-creative scientist. Conversely, the role of the scientist working with nature as the research-and-development team is also important, but neither the scientist nor nature can perform the role of the many participating non-scientists.

THE CLASSROOM FOR THE
CO-CREATIVE NON-SCIENTIST

The classroom for the non-scientist provides a two-part education. First, the non-scientist receives a great deal of his education through the information that is supplied by the scientist when he explains the purpose and principles involved in each new process and program. This information can give the non-scientist a good foundation for understanding the underlying principles of co-creative science solutions. But the non-scientist develops his own personal relationship with nature when he uses the processes, and this is the second way that he learns.

The co-creative processes are designed to connect anyone who uses them directly with nature so that they may form their own team and work together to apply a specific process to a specific situation. Remember that when working with the process, the non-scientist is working with nature. This is the point of the processes: They function as a vehicle for creating a co-creative partnership between a human and nature for the purpose of working together to accomplish a common goal. The process itself represents nature's desire to work with us to address a specific situation.

This partnership between the non-scientist and nature is active and conscious. When a non-scientist chooses to work in a co-creative partnership, he enters his own classroom with nature. But his goal is not to learn how to function as a co-creative research scientist. The non-scientist's goal is to learn how to function as a working partner with nature so that the co-creative processes may be applied appropriately to *every* garden in that person's life.

As the non-scientist, there is a great deal for you to learn, if you wish.

1. You learn when and how to use the processes.

2. You learn how to properly "match" the correct process (or combination of processes) with each situation and how to troubleshoot a problem.

3. You develop clarity in thought, word and action from working with nature.

4. You learn how to ask the right questions and how to ask *good* follow-up questions.

5. You develop the set of communication tools that best suit your own connection with nature.

6. You develop other important tools such as good observation and organization, how to correct mistakes and recognize when you have misunderstood something, and the ability to respond to timing and insight.

7. You have the opportunity to address personal issues that interfere with the quality of how you function in the partnership. As a result, you learn a great deal about your strengths and weaknesses.

8. You learn how to work with nature without manipulating and/or controlling the partnership.

9. From working with nature within the co-creative science structure, you will change the way you think about life and how you approach problems. And you will personally experience nature's intelligence in action.

Your class is less formally set up than the one that is set up for the scientist. However, in its own way, it can be just as intense—and it certainly can be as rewarding and exciting. Especially in the beginning, it can also be frustrating, confusing and mind-boggling, but this is all part of the learning process. The structure for your classes is the co-creative science processes. If you wish to focus on working with nature on your environmental issues, you will be working with the processes in the two *Perelandra Garden Workbook*s. These two books will form the foundation for both your work and learning. If you wish to concentrate on your personal health and your family members' health, you will need to choose one of the co-creative science programs that appeals to you, get the books and material on the subject from Perelandra and start working with the program. Every time you work with one of the programs or processes you will be working with nature directly. And you will have the opportunity for more learning. The more you do the processes, the more you can learn. Your education is structured by nature as much for you personally as the education for the scientist. In short, by using the co-creative science processes in your life, you will step into a new world with nature. At the same time, you will be improving your health, your family's health and the health of your environment. Now, that's not too shabby a deal.

In what areas of our everyday life can co-creative science be applied? Remember in Chapter 1 how nature defined form, nature and a garden. Everything in and around us is form. And according to nature's own definitions, everything in and around us is also nature. For us, nature's universal laws are the prevailing ground rules for all form. Co-creative science applies to every area of our lives. I have specifically pointed out how the scientist develops solutions, but he and nature also develop guidelines of action for preventing imbalances in our health and environment. Add that preventive activity to the solutions to current problems, and the non-scientist has the opportunity to apply co-creative science to any area of his life that he wishes.

Let me give you some examples.

HEALTH

When I refer to health, I am referring not just to *our* health, but the health of our environment, as well. The Perelandra Microbial Balancing Program, a co-creative program that addresses microbial problems both in our health and in the environment, can also be used as a prevention against microbial problems. It is completely natural, has as its underlying foundation the laws of nature and utilizes the notion of balance to achieve solutions to infectious diseases. The following excerpt from the *Perelandra Microbial Balancing Program Manual* will help you understand this particular program, what makes it co-creative and how unique its approach is to the many microbial problems we face today.

> Generally, when we are faced with an infection or an infectious disease, our primary concern is to eliminate the microbe causing the problem. We tend to focus on eradicating the cause so the problem can be solved and health can be restored. For many, the problem with this thinking is that it does not take into consideration that the cause of the problem—microbes—are a population

of live organisms that operate within the laws of nature. The development of drug resistance, which is receiving considerable attention, is only one way that the laws of nature are involved in the interrelationship of microbes and humans. Drug resistance occurs because microorganisms resist any effort to eradicate or kill them. When under siege, they shift into a survival mode because they function within the laws of nature—when attacked, nature does what it must to survive. The weak perish and the strong survive. When bacteria are impacted by antibiotics, they respond by neutralizing the adverse effect of the antibiotic. They do this by mutating. In the short term, most bacteria causing an infection "lose the battle," but the surviving bacteria "win the war." Then the antibiotic no longer threatens their existence. To accomplish this, the bacteria have done nothing more than operate within the laws of nature.

For almost twenty years, I have been working with nature to learn what is required to create a balanced environment within a defined "biosphere." At Perelandra the main focus of this work is the garden. As part of this balancing work, I have had to address the health and well-being of vast and varied populations of microbes (microscopic organisms). They are in the air and soil, and in and on plant systems. Nature has made it clear to me that within any defined biosphere (such as a garden) a balanced microbial population supports that biosphere and enhances its strength. An imbalance in the biosphere will affect the microbes and cause a shift within that population that will enable it to adapt to the imbalance of the biosphere. Conversely, an imbalance within the microbial population will affect the biosphere and force it to shift in order to support the microbial imbalance. Another way of saying this is that the microbial imbalance forces the biosphere to be redefined in a way that accommodates the microbial imbalance. From the perspective of the microbes, they now live in an "appropriately balanced environment." From the perspective of the biosphere, there is now weakness reflecting the microbial imbalance. This usually shows up in specific plants that now have diseases caused by viruses, fungi (pronounced: fun ' ji) and bacteria.

There are three ways to address these interrelated imbalances. One way is to focus on the environment and attempt to restore it to an appropriate balance. This will cause the microbes to shift to accommodate the changed environmental balance. The second way is to focus on the microbes: Address the balance problems in the microbial population, assist that population as we assist the environment to shift to its appropriate balance, and the environment will adjust. The third way is to focus on both the environmental balance and the microbial balance—looking at the problem from both ends. When dealing with environmental and microbial balance, each of these three options for addressing interrelated imbalances must be considered and the appropriate one chosen for the specific situation being addressed.

What does all this about gardens have to do with infectious diseases in humans? The human body is a garden. It is a biosphere that is defined and initiated by the human soul, and it is maintained by humans on both the conscious and unconscious levels. The physical body itself is the biosphere (or form) that is supplied by nature. The health of this biosphere depends on the state of balance and interaction among all elements that make up what is defined as the human being. Microbes are part of those elements. Without them the human biosphere could not function or survive. They are vital to how the body functions. Eliminating them does not shift the body to a greater state of health. Rather, it shifts it to a vastly weakened and endangered state.

There are five major microbial situations that can cause problems for the body biosphere:

1. One microbe enters the human body and causes one infectious disease, such as AIDS or TB.

2. Two different microbes enter the human body and cause two infectious diseases simultaneously, such as AIDS and TB. In this case, AIDS makes the human more susceptible to TB.

3. Many kinds of microbes are released into the body. This occurs when, for example, the appendix ruptures and microorganisms from the intestines are released into the peritoneal cavity.

4. A mixed population of microbes that are a natural part of the body biosphere (for example, in the nasopharyngeal area—the throat—and intestinal tract) become imbalanced.

5. A mixed population of microbes on the surface of the body (such as the arm pits) becomes imbalanced.

As in the Perelandra garden, the key to approaching and working with microbes within and on the human body is balance. The ideal state among an incoming microbe, the microbes that are a natural part of the biosphere and its host environment or biosphere is balance. When an equilibrium among these three elements is maintained, a new natural balance is created and the body does not manifest disease. To obtain this equilibrium, addressing the body directly is not always enough. The balance of the microbes and their relationship to the body's environment need to be considered as well. The Perelandra Microbial Balancing Program was designed by nature to do just this. It applies the principles and processes that have been used successfully in one garden (the Perelandra garden) to the human body garden. And it focuses on one specific, important element within that garden—microbes.

This program may be used in many situations. Obviously, it is to be used any time our health is compromised by a microbial infection. This would include all infections caused by viruses, fungi, bacteria and protozoa. You do not need to know which microbe is causing the infection to use this program. In fact, even if you have been diagnosed by a physician, don't assume the diagnosis is correct. How many times have we heard a physician say, "Well, it's an infection . . . I think it's probably caused by some virus or bacteria." Translated freely, this means it looks like it could be an infection and the physician has no idea what's causing it. In the Microbial Balancing Program, nature easily identifies the imbalance. They're experts at this kind of thing.

In working with this program for myself, I have discovered that I needed it for things that I would not have associated with microbes. For example: I was feeling especially sluggish and my muscles were stiff. I tested that

I needed to do the Microbial Balancing Program for the microbes that were related to this problem. Despite my not understanding the logic behind this, I worked with the program anyway. By the next day I was feeling dramatically better, and by the second day I had more energy and flexibility than I had experienced in months. This example—plus numerous other health issues I have tested—has shown me that, except for well-defined infections, we really don't understand how microbial imbalance affects the human body. So I recommend that you automatically test for the Microbial Balancing Program for any health-related issue. Don't assume anything. If it's not needed, you will find out that it is not needed. Then you can move on to other health alternatives for dealing with the problem.

If you have no obvious health-related issue to test, you may use the Perelandra Microbial Balancing Program to generally balance the microbes that are a part of your body environment (body biosphere). For a general balancing, you will treat the body's entire microbial population as one interactive unit in terms of the relationship of this unit to the body environment. The purpose of this check is to prevent imbalance. By doing a general balancing once a month, you are able to monitor the state of your microbial balance and respond appropriately if it is beginning to reflect a problem. This is especially important during these times when breakdown of the global environment is having an adverse effect on all life systems.

The microbial population within your body is not just affected by your body's balance. It is also influenced by the larger environment outside the body. We are quite aware of the effect the larger environment has on the balance and well-being of our bodies. And it makes sense that whatever affects the body also affects the microbial population. What we don't realize is that the larger environment beyond our body environment also directly affects the microbial population. All we have to do is look at the current worldwide outbreak of bacterial, fungal, viral and protozoan diseases in the environment as well as inside humans to appreciate what I am describing. At the present time, we are not living in environmentally friendly times. Using the Microbial Balancing Program as a preventive measure gives you a vital tool for getting through such times while maintaining a state of balance.

When any biosphere is balanced, it maintains appropriate activity and interaction among all the parts that constitute the biosphere. It naturally and automatically repels anything that does not correspond with or enhance the balance of all that is in the biosphere. This is natural law, and it is also the source of stability and strength inherent in balance. When a biosphere is out of balance, it weakens and becomes vulnerable to and even serves as a magnet for outside elements that support the imbalance. The more a person maintains balance within his body environment, including balance among microbes, the more he will be able to move through life without attracting viruses, fungi, bacteria and protozoa that are currently causing so many serious diseases.

We are quite used to addressing health-related issues by focusing on ourselves. In effect, we ask ourselves what is "wrong" with our body and/or mind that is causing this specific problem. In short, we humans remain in the center position. In terms of the Microbial Balancing Program, the human body is the "host environment" in which the microbes live. This program is focused on the microbes and the state of the host environment (the body environment) as it relates to the microbes. It is the microbes that take center position. For those who have already used the program, this concept was their first eye-opening experience with it. They had to remind themselves often, especially in the beginning, that all of the testing was for what the different microbes needed—not what they (the humans) needed. So be aware that you will most likely be faced with this conceptual shift in the beginning. Don't be afraid to remind yourself often that testing is for the microbes.

Sometimes when working with the program, you will experience physical reactions. If you test that you need the Perelandra Microbial Balancing Program, it means that your microbes are not in balance. This program shifts the microbes and the body environment—as it relates to the microbes—back into balance. This, in turn, affects you personally. For example, you may have a sudden dull headache or mild abdominal pains/cramps that last for five minutes. You might also feel a little light-headed or queasy. Or you might have a sudden flair-up of zits or a bout of itching. A couple of people who had poison ivy several weeks prior to working with the program had a mild recurrence of the rash. In each case the reaction/release was mild, and most reactions disappeared within twenty-four to forty-eight hours. A positive way of looking at this is to realize that whatever is being released would remain within you if you did not use the program. The last thing you want is to incubate a microbial problem in your body. Such an imbalance could lead to serious illness in the future.

Nature tells us that a garden can grow in soil and it can be soil-less. To apply co-creative science to all these gardens, look to the two *Perelandra Garden Workbooks* for the guidelines. As I have said, the laws of nature and the underlying co-creative principles that work for one garden will work for the others. The following are some examples of different gardens taken from letters non-scientists have written to me over the years telling me how the co-creative processes were applied and the results.

ART

Nature supplies the order, organization and life vitality of all the artist's materials. It also helps the artist to function creatively because that function is part of the order, organization and life vitality of the artist's working consciousness. One young woman who applied the *Workbook* processes to her art reported that she experienced significant and exciting changes occurring within her creative process. First was a completely new and comprehensive sense of order. This included the arrangement of tools and furnishings in her studio, what materials and colors to use and which specific pieces she was to work on in conjunction with one another. The improvements in these areas resulted in saving a lot of time, energy and materials. She had been afraid that working with nature in this manner might compromise her free will, personal vision or sense of direction. However, she was surprised to see that these qualities were enhanced and this provided a stronger understanding of her original aim and purpose. She wrote that her greatest challenge was learning to get out of her own way, release control and recognize a better idea when nature provided one. This gave her a deeper understanding of her strengths and weaknesses as an artist and the ability to create more rapidly than she previously thought possible. She also reported that she experienced a lot less head-banging in the process.

ANIMAL HEALING

A woman who had been working with horses for twenty-two years wrote about using the different Perelandra processes in the area of equine medicine. One horse she worked with was impaled on a six- to eight-inch steel bolt that entered into the triceps (shoulder) muscle about seven inches before going downward for another six inches. She used a co-creative nature healing process on the horse right away and the bleeding was immediately slowed to almost nothing. Also, there was never any swelling, which was imperative for the sutures to hold. Later, she worked with nature to determine the loss of "range of motion" in the horse's shoulder and also to see how aggressive she could be while working with the scar tissue and adhesions. After three months of using the co-creative processes, the horse was 98 percent sound.

Another horse had two broken bones in his ankle and was confined to his stall for seven months. She used co-creative processes in deciding which herbs to use for poultices, and which to use for oral treatments. She said she was amazed at the horse's attitude and progress of the injury. After being allowed out of his stall in a restricted area for a limited time, she tested for information about the ankle. She found that the horse needed to be turned out into a larger area so he could walk more to increase the circulation and help the healing process. In just ten months, she tested that the horse had fully recovered and could be ridden.

GARDENING IN SOIL

One person worked with the co-creative Troubleshooting Process to find out what she needed to do to address a severe slug problem in her garden. She did the process that she tested was needed, then went off to work. When she returned that afternoon, the slugs had completely vanished. They remained out of the garden for three days. Then they gradually began to reappear, but she said that they were in balance and eating no more than the plants could handle. Everything in the garden thrived for the rest of the summer.

Another person reported that she had been working with a serious potato bug infestation in her garden. For two years, she tried solving the problem by "relocating" the bugs out of the garden to a wild area that provided plenty for them to eat. This did not solve the problem. On the third year, after noticing the early signs of a very large population on the plants, she used the co-creative science approach and shifted her attitude from relocating the bugs to their achieving a population balance in the garden. In two days the plants that had been covered with the many immature "soft" beetles were virtually beetle-free. She wrote that there remained a most manageable group. And they have maintained the desired balance since.

In another example, a person used co-creative energy processes to clear an area of the garden where nothing would grow. No seeds would sprout and no plants would survive. She did all the processes that she tested were needed for this problem, and during the following week, plants began "reaching" into the empty space and weeds sprouted. From that point on, the area fully supported plant growth.

LEGAL

A woman wrote that she used co-creative processes to support herself through a difficult divorce. In particular, she worked with nature to balance and stabilize herself during a mediation meeting about a joint property dispute she and her former husband were having. As a result of her work, the energy in the meeting room shifted and she participated in the meeting more relaxed than she ever thought possible. The two lawyers efficiently and courteously negotiated the dispute in less than an hour. The attorneys kept remarking that they rarely resolve cases that quickly, with no shouting, no mean stares, and with both parties expressing their desire to be fair. They said more than once that they couldn't believe how smoothly the session went.

TEACHING

A preschool teacher used the *Workbook II* Troubleshooting Process for her class. She had a problem student. He was locked into a power struggle with his mother, could not follow directions, did not participate in group activities and destroyed things. Also, she knew that the room itself had been the setting of a power struggle between a teacher and another student the previous year. That teacher resigned because no solution was found. At the end of her first week in this room with the new "problem" child, the present teacher was experiencing an angry, close-minded reaction to the boy. The testing for the Troubleshooting Process indicated that she needed to do every process on the chart for that room. As she moved through the processes, she could feel the dynamics in the room shift and change. She even needed to do a Geopathic Zone Process on the room. The next day, everything except her conditioned thinking "knew" that things had changed. She reported that old thought patterns were floating on top of a balanced, peaceful and very strong sea. When she walked into her classroom the following week, she discovered the power struggle energy was gone. A clean, focused, useful creative energy was in its place—and the children (including the difficult boy) settled down nicely.

But she wrote that the most incredible thing was the change in her physical energy. She leads an extremely busy life: mother and housewife, plus the preschool responsibilities. She got little sleep and she had hypoglycemia which robbed her of energy if she didn't control what she ate every day. To keep up with her preschool activities, she found it necessary to take a megavitamin, extra protein, spirolina, and kelp plus do a lot of breathing exercises just to maintain an acceptable level of energy. After doing the co-creative processes for her classroom, she found that she did not need to do any of these other things for herself. She didn't need the supplements and her drowsiness didn't show up. She had been fighting her low energy level for over ten years and had tried all kinds of treatments and "answers." Although they helped, it was nothing like the results she had gotten from the co-creative processes that she had used.

A second teacher wrote me about asking nature to assist her in creating an atmosphere in her classroom for maximum learning and healing for the students she worked with and for herself. She said that immediately after setting up with nature and stating her purpose for this classroom, she saw a white light forming a dome-like shape over and above the room and received the insight that this was the light of human evolution. Next, it was joined by the green light of nature and, as she watched, the blue light of teaching appeared. Then the purple (violet) light of transmutation. Next, the yellow light of mental thought. Then the red light of creativity. And finally, a clear orange light of pure and clean emotion. At this point, it dawned on her that a beautiful rainbow had formed. But, as she watched, the lights took form in hundreds of lines. And it became apparent that a grid system was being set into place.

Within the next few days, the population of her students changed. Some children left her classroom and new children were assigned in. Nature's first "directive" to her was to concentrate on teaching the children how to ask for the things that are available to them in this teaching environment. She worked with nature to redesign her class work in order to accommodate the school's requirements for the class according to nature's input. She wrote that she ended up with new and creative ideas for teaching the material. The school formed a teachers group to explore new teaching techniques and asked her to be a part of the group. This allowed her to introduce nature's ideas about the classroom and teaching to her peers.

She did not jeopardize her position by blurting out that she was using nature and co-creative science processes to develop this new teaching. She simply presented the new information as her ideas and in a language that was familiar to the others.

COMPUTERS

Three years ago, a fellow described himself as "the computer nerd who operated as the office wizard" that the other computer users in the business went to when their data evaporated into the ethers of cyberspace. He had an array of tricks he would pull out of his back pocket for healing their fractured files. For this, he received expressions of gratitude and sheer amazement from his co-workers. At the time he wrote the following tale, he had been familiar with the Perelandra processes for years.

> When I'm not keeping bits and bytes in order, I manage the [company] finances. Our bookkeeping is done on computer, based on a fantastic little program called Quicken. It's such a reliable checkbook manager that I took it for granted. I ran disk and tape backups, but more as a formality, and not every day. After all, what were the chances I would actually need them? Well, as I found out a week ago, about 100 percent.
>
> I had just run payroll checks. While they were printing, the nagging thought came to me that I should do a backup. It had been a while since I did one. "OK," I said, "I'll do one just as soon as I'm done with these current transactions." I finally exited Quicken and, remembering another check that needed to be entered, started the program up again. I got the innocent message to the effect that Quicken couldn't read the checkbook

data file. However, it said, don't worry, it will reconstruct the index and we'd be back in business momentarily. This has happened once or twice before, and I know it takes less than a minute to re-do the index.

An hour later, the reconstruction of the index was still going on. But I wasn't worried. Surely, it was just a minor glitch that the good folks at Intuit Software could help me with (they make Quicken). I rummaged around, found the program manual, and dialed the customer support number. I plunged through the voice mail menus and spent twenty minutes on hold, listening to some laid back Palo Alto radio station. The live person who finally came on the line informed me that I had dialed the wrong support number. He very graciously offered to connect me to the right number. I was soon back in the voice mail twilight zone, listening to more music from Palo Alto.

I gave up on the customer support idea. I figured the easiest thing would be to restore the data file from my most recent backup (three weeks old, I'm ashamed to admit), and then re-enter the transactions from my paper trail of receipts and deposit slips. This was when I discovered that my normally reliable disk backup had gone south. Now I was sweating a little, but not really worried, since I had a tape backup that was five weeks old. It would just mean a little reconstructive work on my part to get the file back in shape. Since it was late in the day, I closed shop and left the office, confident that I would run the tape restore in the morning, and all would be well. The next morning, I loaded the tape into the drive, commanded it to restore my lost file and . . .

Nothing! The tape backup was bad as well! As some yawning chasm started opening up in the pit of my stomach, my mind was wondering about the odds of two normally reliable backup procedures failing at the same time. I calculated them to be pretty high indeed.

Full blown panic was huffing and puffing and trying to blow my mental house down, but I did my best to remain calm and scrape the bottom of my cerebral cavity for new ideas. It was slim pickings. I was even ready to get on the phone to Palo Alto and spend the morning listening to more music, though I doubted that the Intuit gurus could really get my data back at this point. That's when I got the idea to ask nature for help!

I connected with the deva of the computer finance program and asked for help or intuition. A few minutes later, I got the hit to open Quicken without the payroll module and allow it to reconstruct the index that way. It worked. I had all my data back in less than a minute. The clouds parted, birds sang and I said, "Well, I'll be (unprintable). It worked!" I thanked nature for its help.

I learned several things from this experience. First, I now run *three* distinct backup procedures and have tested each one to make sure they actually work reliably. I also now keep a paper copy of all transactions. Second, and more important, I've learned how helpful it is to include nature as a partner in my computer work, not only in disaster recovery but in organizing my procedures to make disaster unlikely. I have a clearer sense of how my computer and finance work is just another type of garden, subject to the same co-creative principles as the Perelandra garden.

BOOK WRITING AND BOOK PRODUCTION

I guess I don't need to tell you that I use co-creative science processes throughout every area of my life. Of course, I use co-creative principles for all of the Perelandra research and development. After all, it would be tough for a co-creative scientist to function otherwise. But I also run the Perelandra business using the same principles. And my staff incorporates co-creative processes in production, construction, organization, office management and business meetings. I especially enjoy using co-creative science when I am writing a book. In Chapter 1, I pointed out that since a book is form, it is also nature. I work with the deva of each book for all of the writing sessions and for the design and production elements, as well. We prepare the camera-ready copy for the printer in-house, so we have full control over what our published books say and how they are designed. I am what is known in the trade as a "first-draft" writer. That is, I'm able to lay down such a solid first draft that all I need to do is put the manuscript through the copyediting stage (I have a terrific copyeditor) and move it through the rest of the production stages. There are no rewrites for my manuscripts. I'd like to say I am extraordinarily talented as a writer, but, quite frankly, my success in this area centers around the help I get from working with nature throughout the entire book process.

LAND AND ENERGY

Nature said that energy is just form that we can't perceive with our five senses. All form operates within the same overall universal principles. (That's why the co-creative science processes that are developed in a vegetable garden can be equally applied to other arenas.) Energy that is out of balance has as much of an ecological impact as sulfur emissions, toxic waste and low-level radiation. It's just that with energy pollution we can't see it, so we tend not to address it. In actuality, most folks don't even know that their environment is deteriorating just as rapidly from energy pollution as from five-senses pollution. We are directly affected by energy pollution in fundamental ways. For example:

I knew a fellow who was going through a particularly strange and vitriolic divorce. He was completely caught off guard when his wife suddenly ended the marriage and moved out in a somewhat dramatic manner. What was strange was that she kept returning when he wasn't around to dig up plants and perennials in all of the gardens and beds. He said that whenever he returned, the property felt like something had been ripped out of it. He also said that he felt that she was acting out her anger on the land. When he heard about the work I was doing at Perelandra, he asked me if there was something I could do that would be helpful to the land.

I worked from a well-drawn map of their property which showed the placement of the woods, swamp, fields, house, driveway and gardens. It was an isolated piece of land—about thirty-five acres—that was way in the country. I set up with nature and tested for the processes this land needed. One process that I tested was needed was the Battle Energy Release Process. After going through its steps, it was clear to me that part of the battle energy that was released was the divorce. In fact, there was so much battle energy activity around the house and garden areas that I suggested to him that he do a little research and find out the history of the house regarding previous owners.

He got back to me several weeks later. It seems that the house had remained empty for a number of years prior to their purchasing and restoring it. But he was able to find out that the family who had owned the house before them had gone through a divorce that had exactly the same dynamics: the wife left suddenly and unexpectedly, the process was especially vitriolic and she kept returning to rip up the gardens.

We don't know what the history was prior to that couple. But I can say that the energy that was released by them around this divorce didn't just dissipate into nothingness. It had to go somewhere. When I developed the Battle Energy Release Process with nature, I learned that nature absorbs unprocessed, emotional energy which, in turn, buffers us from being constantly battered by an environment of everyone's emotional releases. What also happens is that the molecular makeup of the form alters to accommodate the new energy. There is a universal principle that nature repeats to me over and over: like attracts like. When you have an environment that has contained within it the energy elements of particular human action and interaction, that environment then supports this kind of action.

I'm not saying that the history of the land caused these two people to divorce. Most likely, they would have divorced anyway. But what the land did do was enhance and support those feelings and actions that had already been played out at least once in this house. Without realizing it, the two present owners automatically adjusted their thinking and actions in a manner that was supported by the energy makeup of their biosphere. Their personal options in moving through the separation and divorce became limited.

The energy-process work that I did appropriately released the various energy elements that were part of their biosphere that did not enhance balance. By the way, once I completed this work, the wife no longer returned to dig up the gardens.

INNER-CITY HOUSING

Here's another example of an environment's balance affecting how we conduct our lives. I have a friend who ran a firm that trained and assisted inner-city project residents to take over the management and eventual ownership of their own buildings. These types of projects are usually one step away from total collapse in every way. The residents must be taught a range of skills from financial management to repair and maintenance. On the whole, my friend's firm was recognized in the community as being a successful alternative to inner-city housing problems. But the success was often hard fought.

Well, as I listened to my friend describe the problems, I could tell that the residents they were working with were perfectly capable of learning the necessary skills and taking over the project management. They were not stupid people. But her firm was meeting with all kinds of resistance from these people. In some cases, it was like trying to pull their feet out of tar. All of the projects were in areas of the city that were run down and low income. There was a high crime rate and a lot of drug dealing. And these kinds of problems had existed in those areas for many years.

I kept saying to her that she had a problem with how the people and the building and its land were interacting. On the one hand, her firm was attempting to assist the people to make a major step forward in how they lived their lives. On the other hand, the buildings they lived in and the land upon which the buildings sat were physically supporting the very things the people were trying to move away from. It was as if a totally sane person was locked up in our worst nightmare of a mental institution and was not only expected to continue to act sane but also to make significant progress in a new discipline. It's not fair to ask or expect someone to function in exceptional ways under these conditions. My friend had to change the balance of the environment so that it enhanced and supported the new.

The residents had already committed themselves to changing and taking charge of their situation. It was clear from their actions that, as they opened up to the intent of their commitment, they became more sensitive. But their ability to move forward became more hampered. The personal issues they needed to face in order to make these changes were magnified by the emotional energies that were already present in their environment. Their personal difficulties became magnets to these energies—like attracting like. It was doubly difficult for the residents to personally change because what they were attempting to move away from was constantly being energized by their environment.

To be honest, my friend thought I was nuts—well, mildly nuts—when I told her what I thought needed to be done. At best, I was obsessing and trying to shove this nature business off on her. But because she was my friend, I took the liberty to push a little and to keep chipping away at her. Eventually, I said just the right words and she finally heard them. She then understood—conceptually—that these people were being held back because of all the energy patterns that were part of their environment. She armed herself with the necessary Perelandra material and went back to the city to try working with co-creative science.

I got a call from her a couple of weeks later. She reported that she did three energy processes at her office first. She told no one what she had done. Immediately, people began relating to one another differently. She needed to make some difficult personnel changes anyway, and the process resulted in a smaller, tighter, more efficient team. She also needed to reorganize her office, and that process also worked in ways that defied reason.

She already knew kinesiology. So she had the tool in place for making contact and working with nature in this new partnership. She used the simple yes/no format with nature. She was instructed on how to set up their work together, make small models of all of the projects her firm had contracts for and to gather small soil samples from the grounds of each project. She was then to place the soil samples in the models. From her office, she was to work with nature to balance and stabilize each of the projects.

She worked with one huge project first. It had a total of fifteen buildings. She collected a soil sample from each of the buildings' grounds, plus she was told to put a sample from the fifteen grounds into the centrally located common-ground area in the model. She worked with nature to do the various needed processes in the order they were to be done and for the specific areas for which they tested they were needed, and then she balanced and stabilized each building and its land.

Whatever was needed for this, she just dropped a small amount onto the soil sample in the model.

Various things happened within days of her work. For one thing, she had to meet with the local electric company to ask for an extension regarding funding so that energy conservation training could be extended throughout the entire project. This was important because as the people moved into the newly renovated apartments, they had to assume the energy bills. Up until then, these bills had always been included in the rent. Without the training, the tenants would experience severe money traumas from the high energy bills. My friend was anticipating a real problem with the electric company—in fact, she was expecting a confrontation. Instead, they informed her, as she walked in the door, that they were giving both her and this project an extension. Kiss that confrontation goodbye. Not only this, but her firm also got, at the same time, the final approval for the increased training funds from the government *after* the government had already rejected the funding in writing. They had reversed themselves and decided that the funding would come out of capital expenses and that it was considered "an investment in the future."

Then about five days after she did the energy work, there was an open house at the project. She said it was great. For the first time, the residents helped support the existing management in the new direction, and the owners acknowledged and supported this new direction, recognizing the residents as the future owners of the building complex

Since that time, that particular project moved forward in leaps and bounds. The residents, along with the owners and management, came up with the idea of using the common ground to establish the first inner-city plant and tree nursery and to work together to make it a money-making venture. The existing owner had already contracted a landscape architect and nurseryman to work with the residents and help set up the program. In short, this particular housing project was well on its way to becoming a model program.

My friend worked with nature on the other projects her firm was responsible for and she has seen dramatic results. She's operating in the "straight world" and isn't talking about what she is doing, of course. She's letting the results speak for themselves and she is only answering the questions that people are asking. She also worked on a way that this nature information and work can be taught to the residents without infringing on their personal belief systems. Ideally, it would be best if the residents took over the responsibility of maintaining the energy balance of their own environment.

Her work was so successful and she became so recognized for it that she now works on the national level. She still hasn't told anyone what she is doing with those models.

Like attracts like. Several months after beginning her work with co-creative science, my friend attended a conference in Switzerland. While there, she got into a conversation with a fellow that led to sharing information about her nature work. He ended up asking her to help him and his group clear out, balance and stabilize a large building they had been given to convert into an international peace studies center. It had once been part of a Nazi concentration camp during World War II.

And what does nature say about all of this? The following session with the Overlighting Deva of Planet Earth applies equally for co-creative scientists and non-scientists alike. Read this session with our new understanding of the words "nature," "form" and "garden" and what nature intelligence means when it uses these words.

OVERLIGHTING DEVA OF PLANET EARTH

I have looked forward to this moment, to the opportunity to add to the effort being made through the vehicle of this book. I am the overlighting consciousness of the planet upon which you live. I have been referred to as "Gaia" by many. I would like to give you insight into the physical evolution of the planet as seen from my perspective.

All that exists in the solar system of which planet Earth is a part and in the countless realms and dimensions beyond is presently moving through a major shift. Some of you refer to this as the movement from the Piscean era to the Aquarian era. Earth is not an out-of-step planet struggling within an in-step universe to reach the level of perfection that surrounds it. It is quite a common thing for humans on Earth to perceive themselves as lesser, behind in development and out of step. This very notion is what one may call "Piscean" in its dynamic. It sets up the planet and those souls who are choosing to experience the lessons of form in a parent/child situation —the universe being the parent, the planet and its inhabitants being the child. It was an important dynamic of the Piscean era, this continuous sense of the child striving and moving forward toward the all-knowing parent, and a dynamic which was played out in one way or another on every level of interaction on Earth. The notion of the parent served as the impetus to keep the child moving forward in the hope that one day, after much work and growth, the child would attain the peer position with the parent.

The parent/child notion has not been exclusive to Earth. It is a dynamic that has been part of reality on all other dimensions and levels. And as already stated, it has been an important dynamic of the Piscean era for the souls on all levels to come to grips with in whatever manner needed. I point this out to emphasize that Earth is part of an ever-evolving whole and not the bastard child of that whole.

The important lesson to be integrated into the picture of reality from the parent/child dynamic was the conscious, personal dedication of the individual to move forward. The parent dynamic stood before the child within all and encouraged those vital steps forward toward the perceived notion of perfection represented by the parent. It served to weave into the individual's fabric of life that sense of constant forward motion and the knowing that its resulting change led to something better and greater.

Although the parent/child dynamic has been a tangible force that has permeated the levels of reality during the Piscean era, the actual fact of every individual being the child seeking to move toward a parent has been illusion. It is how a Piscean dynamic was translated into a workable reality. An impulse was released within all levels of reality some two thousand years ago, and each individual receiving this impulse translated it into an understandable, tangible concept. The main thrust of the overall translation on planet Earth has been the parent/child dynamic. There has been, in fact, no parent outside and beyond who has enticed and encouraged the children forward. Just as the child is within all, so, too, is the parent. But in order to develop the tools they needed to move forward in confidence, individuals needed to establish that sense of the all-knowing parent standing before them in the unknown, ready to catch, comfort and receive them as they take those shaky steps forward.

I have not forgotten to address the planet Earth. I needed to lay the foundation for you to understand how the principles presented in this book fit into the larger picture—and that includes Earth.

When the parent/child impulse was released throughout reality, it was received not only by individual human souls, but by the planet as a whole. I have stated that the impulse was sounded on all levels of reality. In order for there to be harmonious evolution, there must be a sense of tandem movement within the whole. The impulse was received and seated within planet Earth, which, in turn, stabilized the seating of the impulse within individuals. Now, as human souls translated that impulse into the workable parent/child dynamic, that translation itself seated into the planet and its various natural forms, thus modifying the original impulse to conform to the translation. This is natural law—form conforming to the energy within. It is a necessary part of the support system between spirit and matter. One cannot have the spirit reflecting one reality seated within a form energized by another reality. It would be as if two horses were hitched to one another but pulling in opposite directions. There would be no chance of forward movement. So, form must conform in order for there to be mutual support and evolution between matter and spirit.

To broaden this picture even more, let me say that the impulse and the translation of the impulse (as with all the Piscean impulses and their translations) placed the individuals and the planet squarely and solidly into the evolutionary picture of its universe as a whole—not out of step with it. The planet has been an active participant in understanding and working with what we might call "contemporary issues," for the issues have been the same throughout reality; only the translations have differed. It has been vital that the specific parent/child translation, for example, be fully explored and understood by those on Earth so that the resulting knowledge could be made accessible to the whole. Likewise, other translations of the very same impulse have been made accessible to the whole and have been received at various times throughout the Piscean era by individuals and the intelligences of nature on Earth.

Now a new set of impulses has been sounded throughout reality, and they are the impulses referred to by some as "Aquarian." All of reality has moved into a period of transition. The impulses are in the process of being fully seated in and translated everywhere. On Earth, we have full reception of the initial Aquarian impulses. They are seated well within the planet and are now serving the shift of those living on the planet from Piscean to Aquarian.

If you have followed my train of thought, you will realize that with the planet itself holding the Aquarian impulses, all that exists on the planet and all its individuals are not only receiving the similar impulses but the impetus and support from the planet to change, as well. This means that those translations and the resulting systems and procedures from the old simply will not function as smoothly in the present. The soul energy of the planet has shifted and no longer corre- lates with the old form translations that exist on its surface. And very shortly, you will see a rapid deterioration of all that has worked so well in the past. New translations are required. New systems and procedures. The planet is already holding the new impulses.

The co-creative gardening processes as presented in the Perelandra Garden Workbooks are a translation of the new. They work because they once again align spirit and matter with parallel intent and purpose. In this case, one could say we have a double alignment. We have the spirit of the human translating impulse into new form and action, and we have the connection of the spirit of the human with the new im- pulses contained within the planet around him. As you incor- porate these translations into thought and action, you will see evidence of effortless change all around you. As already stated, this is because the intent of spirit and the intent of matter are realigning and once again moving in tandem.

This brings me back to the parent/child notion of the Pis- cean era. One of the translations of this dynamic from hu- mans has been in the arena of nature. That is, humans have tended to look at nature either as the parent looking at a child in need of discipline, or the child seeking beneficial aid and assistance from the powerful and all-knowing parent. In essence, humans have translated the parent/child dynamic in nature as either manipulation or worship. Both translations were working, viable frameworks for learning, but they are both no longer workable. For humans to continue attempting to respond and to act within these two mindsets is wreaking havoc on the planet itself.

With the Aquarian dynamic, the parent/child is uniting as one balanced, integrated force within the individual. It is the uniting of the universal wisdom contained within all and the absolute knowledge that in order to have full, conscious access to that universal wisdom, one must continue to move forward in the learning and changing mode. The parent and child come together in balanced partnership.

The co-creative garden translates this fundamental Aquarian dynamic into the arena of nature. Human and nature come together in conscious, equal partnership, both functioning from a position of wisdom and change. Wherever such a garden is initiated, it will immediately sound a note outward into the universe and inward into the core of the planet, the very soul of the planet, that the shift from Piscean to Aquarian dynamics within that nature arena is in the process of change. And immediately, the evolving intent of the garden will be aligned with the prevailing universal flow and the corresponding planetary impulses, one buttressing from above, the other buttressing from below within the planet. The result will be forward motion in tandem—the gardener in tandem with his planet and his universe. With this massive support, it is no wonder the co-creative garden works.

Allow me to give you another insight. The Aquarian impulses are already seated within the planet. Visualize, if you will, the planet as a container of these impulses—energy held beneath the Earth's surface. This energy is seated within the very soul of the planet, seated within its heart. It is there to be released and integrated into all levels of life on the planet.

Now, picture one, small co-creative garden on the planet's surface. See it as a window into the interior of the planet, into its soul. As the gardener works to align this garden to the new dynamics, watch the window open and the energy contained within the core of the planet gently gravitate to and release through the window. Feel the sense of relief and freedom within the Earth's core as the energy moves upward and out. And watch the actions and the form on the Earth's surface suddenly shift to reflect the impact of the heart energy that has now surfaced. That which exists on the surface has begun to connect to and integrate with the heart and soul of the planet, which, in turn, is fully aligned with the heart and soul force of the universe. As each person opens the window through the framework of the co-creative garden to the heart and soul energy of the planet, Earth will experience what a human experiences when he consciously shifts his perceptions and suddenly releases the heart energy he holds deep within—balance and peace.

It is not enough to move about the planet in a state of benevolent love for it. This human state alone will not create the passageways through which the heart energy of the planet is allowed to release. It must be accomplished through the state of the human mind, human consciousness, combined with parallel and appropriate action. Once released, this heart energy from the planet will permeate all living reality upon its surface and support the evolutionary process of the planet and its inhabitants in tandem movement with the universe into the Aquarian era.

I fully understand that I am aligning deep planetary change and universal movement with the actions of one gar-

dener tending one small garden. This is precisely what I mean to do. One need not wait for group consensus in such matters. One need only move forward, sound the note for change, and follow that intonation with parallel action. Each gardener, in the role of the Knower, shall hold the seed to his heart and shall plant this seed in the earth. The fruit of this plant shall be the winged and shafted Sun above his head, and a new kingdom shall be grounded on Earth. This I can promise you. This is what awaits you.

Appendix A

Kinesiology Testing

Kinesiology is another name for muscle testing. If you want to get information from nature, all you have to do is ask simple yes/no questions that will give you the information you seek. (By "simple," I mean questions that can have only one answer, not two questions in one sentence, each requiring its own answer.) Nature will project a "yes" or "no" into your electrical system and you will then be able to discern the answer by kinesiology testing your electrical system.

For those of you who have never heard of such a thing but would like to try it, I am reprinting the information on developing kinesiology testing from the *Perelandra Garden Workbook* (second edition).

KINESIOLOGY:
THE TOOL FOR TESTING

Kinesiology is simple. Anybody can do it because it uses your electrical system and your muscles. If you are alive, you have these two things. I know that sounds smart-mouthed of me, but I've learned that sometimes people refuse to believe that anything can be so simple. So they create a mental block —only "sensitive types" can do this, or only women can do it. It's just not true. Kinesiology happens to be one of those simple things in life just waiting around to be learned and used by everyone.

I don't mean to intimidate you, but small children can learn to do kinesiology in about five minutes. It is mainly because it never occurred to them that they couldn't do it. If I tell them they have an electrical system, they don't argue with me about it—they just get on with the business of learning how to do simple testing. Actually, I do mean to intimidate you. Your first big hurdle will be whether or not you believe you have a viable electrical system that is capable of being tested. Here's a good test. Place a hand mirror under your nose. If you see breath marks, you have a strong electrical system. (If you don't see breath marks, call your local emergency rescue squad—you're in trouble.) Now you can get on with learning how to use kinesiology!

If you've ever been to a chiropractor or holistic physician experienced in muscle testing, you've experienced kinesiology. The doctor tells you to stick out your arm and resist his pressure. It feels like he is trying to push your arm down after he has told you not to let him do it. Everything is going fine, and then all of a sudden he presses and your arm falls down like a floppy fish no matter how hard you try to keep it up. That is using kinesiology.

Simply stated, the body has within it and surrounding it an electrical network or grid. If anything impacts your electrical system that does not maintain or enhance your health and your body's balance, your muscles, when having physical pressure applied, are unable to hold their strength. (Muscle power is directly linked to the balance of the electrical system.) In other words, if pressure is applied to an individual's extended arm while his body's electrical system is being adversely affected, the muscles will weaken and the arm will not be able to resist the pressure. The circuits of the electrical system are overloaded or have short-circuited, causing a weakening of that system. However, if pressure is applied while his electrical system is being positively affected, the circuits remain strong, balanced and capable of fully functioning throughout the body. The muscles will remain strong, the person will easily resist and the arm will hold its position.

This electrical/muscular relationship is a natural part of the human system. It is not mystical or magical. Kinesiology is the established method for reading the body's balance through the balance of the electrical system at any given moment.

When working in a co-creative partnership, nature answers your yes/no questions by projecting a positive energy or a negative energy—whichever is appropriate—into the electrical circuit that you have created by your fingers especially for the kinesiology testing. The "yes" or "no" that nature projects registers in this one electrical connection and not throughout your entire electrical system. The special connection created by your fingers allows you to use the kinesiology technique without adversely impacting your electrical system or your body's balance. Only one circuit is being used, and this circuit is artificially created by you for the testing and is not a part of the normal function of the electrical system throughout your body. The answer you are able to discern through the testing is from nature. It is not an answer that has been concocted by you.

If you have ever experienced muscle testing, you probably participated in the above-described, two-person operation.

You provided the extended arm, and the other person provided the pressure. Although efficient, this can sometimes be
cumbersome when you want to test something on your own.
Arm pumpers have the nasty habit of disappearing right when
you need them most. So you will be learning to self-test—no
arm pumpers needed.

KINESIOLOGY SELF-TESTING STEPS

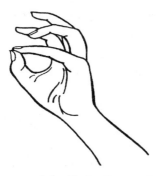

1. THE CIRCUIT FINGERS. If
you are right-handed: Place your
left hand palm up. Connect the
tip of your left thumb with the
tip of the left little finger (not
your index finger). If you are
left-handed: Place your right
hand palm up. Connect the tip of
your right thumb with the tip of
your right little finger. By connecting your thumb and little
finger, you have closed an electrical circuit in your hand, and
it is this circuit you will use for testing.

Before going on, look at the position you have just formed
with your hand. If your thumb is touching the tip of your
index or first finger, laugh at yourself for not being able to
follow directions, and change the position to touch the tip of
the thumb with the tip of the little or fourth finger. Most
likely this will not feel at all comfortable to you. If you are
feeling a weird sense of awkwardness, you've got the first
step of the test position! In time, the hand and fingers will adjust to being put in this position and it will feel fine.

Circuit fingers can touch tip to tip, finger pad to finger pad, or thumb resting on top of the little finger's nail. Women with long nails need not impale themselves.

2. THE TEST FINGERS. To test the circuit (the means by which you will apply pressure to yourself), place the thumb and index finger of your other hand inside the circle you have created by connecting your thumb and little finger. The thumb and index finger should be right under your thumb and your little finger, touching them. Don't try to make a circle with your test fingers. They are just placed 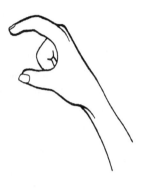 inside the circuit fingers that do form a circle. It will look as if the circuit fingers are resting on the test fingers.

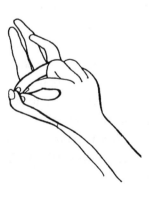

3. POSITIVE RESPONSE. Keeping this position, ask yourself a yes/no question in which you already know the answer to be yes. ("Is my name _____?") Once you've asked the question, press your circuit fingers together, keeping the tip-to-tip position. *Using the same amount of pressure,* try to pull apart the circuit fingers with your test fingers. Press the lower thumb against the upper thumb, and the lower index finger against the upper little finger.

The action of your test fingers will look like scissors separating as you apply pressure to your circuit fingers. The motion of the test fingers is horizontal. Don't try to pull your test fingers vertically up through your circuit fingers. This action sometimes works but it is not as reliable as the horizontal scissors action.

The circuit position described in step 1 corresponds to the position you take when you stick your arm out for the physician. The testing position in step 2 is in place of the physician or other convenient arm pumper. After you ask the yes/no question and you press your circuit fingers tip-to-tip, that is equal to the doctor saying, "Resist my pressure." Your circuit fingers now correspond to your outstretched, stiffened arm. Trying to pull apart those fingers with your testing fingers is equal to the doctor pressing down on your arm.

If the answer to the question is positive (if your name is what you think it is!), you will not be able to easily pull apart the circuit fingers. The electrical circuit will hold, your muscles will maintain their strength, and your circuit fingers will not separate. You will feel the strength in that circuit.

IMPORTANT: Be sure the amount of pressure holding the circuit fingers together is equal to the amount of your testing fingers pressing against them. Also, don't use a pumping action in your test fingers when applying pressure to your circuit fingers. Use an equal, steady and continuous pressure.

Play with this a bit. Ask a few more yes/no questions that have positive answers. Now, I know it is going to seem that if you already know the answer to be "yes," you are probably "throwing" the test. That's reasonable, but for the time being, until you get a feeling for what the positive response feels like, you're going to need to deliberately ask yourself questions with positive answers.

While asking questions, if you are having trouble sensing the strength of the circuit, apply a little more pressure. Or consider that you may be applying too much pressure and pull back some. You don't have to break or strain your fingers for this; just use enough pressure to make them feel alive, connected and alert.

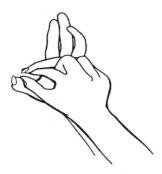

4. NEGATIVE RESPONSE. Once you have a clear sense of the positive response, ask yourself a question that has a negative answer. Again press your circuit fingers together and, using equal pressure, press against the circuit fingers with the test fingers. This time the electrical circuit will break and the circuit fingers will weaken and separate. Because the electrical circuit is broken, the muscles in the circuit fingers do not have the power to easily hold the fingers together. In a positive state the electrical circuit holds, and the muscles have the power to keep the two fingers together.

How much your circuit fingers separate depends on your personal style. Some people's fingers separate a lot. Other's barely separate at all. Mine separate about a quarter of an inch. Some people's fingers won't separate at all, but they'll definitely feel the fingers weaken when pressure is applied during a "no" answer. Give yourself time and let your personal style develop naturally.

Also, if you are having a little trouble feeling anything, do your testing with your forearms resting in your lap. This way you won't be using your muscles to hold up your arms while trying to test.

Play with negative questions a bit, and then return to positive questions. Get a good feeling for the strength between your circuit fingers when your electrical system is balanced and the weakness when it is short-circuited or imbalanced. You can even ask yourself (your own system) for a positive response and then, after testing, ask for a negative response. ("Give me a positive response." Test. "Give me a negative response." Test.) You will feel the positive strength and the negative weakness. In the beginning, you may feel only a slight difference between the two. With practice, that difference will become more pronounced. For now, it is just a matter of trusting what you have learned—and practicing.

Don't forget the overall concept behind kinesiology. What enhances our body, mind and soul makes us strong. Together, our body, mind and soul create an environment that, when balanced, is strong and solid. If something enters that environment and challenges the balance, the environment is weakened. That strength or weakness first registers in the electrical system, and it can be discerned through the muscle-testing technique—kinesiology.

KINESIOLOGY TIPS

If you are having trouble feeling a positive and negative response in the circuit fingers, try switching hands—the circuit fingers become the test fingers and vice versa. Most people who are right-handed have this particular electrical circuitry that is used in kinesiology in their left hand. Left-handers generally have the circuitry in their right hand. But sometimes a right-hander has the circuitry in the right hand and a left-hander has it in the left hand. You may be one of those people. If you are ambidextrous, choose the circuit hand that gives you the clearest responses. Before deciding which to use, give yourself a couple of weeks of testing using one hand as the circuit hand to get a good feel for its responses before trying the other hand.

If you have an injury such as a muscle sprain in either hand or arm, don't try to learn kinesiology until you have healed. Kinesiology is muscle testing, and a muscle injury will interfere with the testing—and the testing will interfere with the healing of the muscle injury.

Also, when first learning kinesiology, do yourself a favor and set aside some quiet time to go through the instructions and play with the testing. Trying to learn this while riding the New York subway during evening rush hour isn't going to give you the break you need. But once you have learned it, you will be able to test all kinds of things while riding the subway.

Sometimes I meet people who are trying to learn kinesiology and are not having much luck. They have gotten frustrated, decided this isn't for them, and have gone on to try to learn another means of testing. Well, I'll listen to them explain what they did, and before they know it, I've verbally tricked them with a couple of suggestions about their testing, which they try, and they begin feeling kinesiology for the first time—a strong "yes" and a clear "no." The problem wasn't kinesiology. Everyone, as I have said, has an electrical system. The problem was that they wanted to learn it so much that they became overly anxious and tense—they blocked.

So, since you won't have me around to trick you, I suggest that if you suspect you're blocking, turn your focus for several days, even a couple of weeks, to something completely different. Then trick yourself. When you care the least about whether or not you learn kinesiology, start playing with it again. Approach it as if it were a game. *Then* you'll feel the strength and weakness in the fingers.

If you're still not getting a satisfactory "yes" and "no" after several weeks of trying, ask nature to help you learn and develop kinesiology. In fact, it can help you unjam the logs around this issue. Simply direct your focus to nature (nature intelligence) and state that you would like it to help you learn to do kinesiology testing. Also state that you would like to feel a clear positive and negative response in your testing. Then walk away from trying to test for the rest of the day and return to it in a day or two. Read the kinesiology steps again and practice the testing. This time, pay attention to any intuitive "hits" you might receive about the testing and play with the information. Now you'll have success with feeling "yes" and "no."

TROUBLESHOOTING KINESIOLOGY

Suppose the testing has been working fine, and then suddenly you can't get a clear result (what I call a "definite maybe") or get no result at all. Check the following:

1. SLOPPY TESTING. You press apart the fingers *before* applying pressure between the circuit fingers. This happens most often when we have been testing for awhile and become over-confident or do the testing too quickly. I think it happens to all of us from time to time and serves to remind us to keep our attention on the matter at hand. (Excuse the pun.)

Especially in the beginning, start a kinesiology session by "warming up"—that is, feel a few positive and negative responses. Ask yourself some of those obvious questions. Or simply say several times, "Let me feel a positive." (Test.) "Let me feel a negative." (Test.) This warm-up will remind you what positive and negative responses feel like before you start.

2. EXTERNAL DISTRACTIONS. Trying to test in a noisy or active area can cause you to lose concentration. The testing will feel unsure or contradict itself if you double-check the results. Often, simply moving to a quiet, calm spot and concentrating on what you are doing will be just what's needed for successful testing.

3. FOCUS OR CONCENTRATION. Even in a quiet spot, one's mind may wander and the testing will feel fuzzy, weak or contradictory. It is important to concentrate throughout the process. Check how you are feeling. If you're tired, I suggest you not try to test until you have rested a bit. And if you have to go to the bathroom, do it. That little situation is a sure concentration-destroyer.

4. THE QUESTION ISN'T CLEAR. A key to kinesiology is asking a simple yes/no question, not two questions in one,

each having a possible yes/no answer. If your testing isn't working, first check your hand positions. Next, review your question, and make sure you are asking only one question. And, while you're asking a question, don't think ahead to the next question! Your fingers won't know which to answer.

5. MATCH YOUR INTENT WITH HOW YOU WORD YOUR QUESTION. If you are prone to saying, "Oh, I didn't mean to say that!" when you talk to others, this might be an area you need to work on.

A woman at one of our workshops asked me about some strange answers she had gotten about what to feed her cat. She had asked, "What kinds of food would make my cat happy?" She got some pretty weird answers like chocolate, catnip, steak. . . . I pointed out that she probably asked the wrong question. She meant to ask nature what foods would make her cat healthy. She was a little surprised. She thought that this was the question she had originally asked. In short, her question and her intent did not match.

6. YOU MUST WANT TO ACCEPT THE RESULTS OF THE TEST. If you enter a kinesiology test not wanting to "hear" the answer, for whatever reason, you can override the test with your emotions and your will. This is true for conventional situations as well. If you really don't want something to work for you, it won't work. That's our personal power dictating the outcome.

Also, if you are trying to do testing during a situation that is especially emotional for you, that deeply stirs your emotions, or if you are trying to ask a question in which you have a strong, personal investment in the answer, I suggest that you not test until you are calmer or get some emotional distance from the situation. During such times, you are walking a very fine line between a clear test and a test that your desires are overriding. Kinesiology as a tool is not the issue here. It is the condition or intent of the tester.

7. CONTRADICTORY RESULTS. If your testing has been going along just fine and you suddenly begin to get contradictory or "mushy" test results, consider that this may not be a good day for you to do this particular work. Or you may need to drink water. If you are dehydrated, your electrical system will feel weak during kinesiology testing.

A NOTE ON CLARITY

If you are having difficulty wording a simple yes/no question, consider this an important issue to be faced and something worth spending time to rectify. You have not simply stumbled upon a glitch in your quest to use kinesiology. You have also stumbled upon a glitch in the communication between you and nature. This is not as serious a situation with non-scientists because they have all the steps and procedures to the processes already set for them and they need only do simple testing with nature. But, even as a non-scientist working with co-creative science, you will need to know how to ask some questions. However, for the co-creative scientist, this is a critical situation. You must be able to ask clear and concise questions. You must also develop a good flexibility around questions if you wish to work with nature well. If you can't even clearly phrase the question, you can't expect an answer. I have met people who cannot articulate a question. In a workshop they will attempt to ask me something and I can't figure out what they are asking—nor can anyone else in the workshop. Usually it turns out that they are frustrated because they can't get any clarity in their own life and are trying to ask me what to do about it.

For those of you who find yourselves in this boat, you have a terrific opportunity to turn that around and develop internal order by learning how to articulate a simple yes/no question. If you do this, you not only develop the tool of kinesiology, you also develop clarity for communicating with nature—and everyone else around you.

If you need to develop yourself in this area, I recommend that you initially devote your attention to learning to ask simple questions and not worry about receiving answers. When you need to ask someone a question, take time to consider what you really want to ask and how it can be most clearly and efficiently worded. It helps to write down the question. In this way, you can visually see your words. If they don't convey what you want to express, play with the wording. Keep doing this until you feel those words accurately and concisely communicate what you wish to ask. Then go to that person and ask the question. Notice the difference in the quality of how the person answers you. Your clarity will inspire similar clarity in the response.

Quite often, that frustrating inner confusion we experience exists because we have not had an acceptable framework for the development of mental ordering. Learning to ask questions gives the mind something tangible to work with and, in the process, you learn mind-word-and-mouth coordination.

You'll find that as you develop the ability to clearly articulate a simple question, your inner fog will begin to lift, which in turn will automatically begin to lift your outer fog. Another point: It also will be helpful to focus on your ability to ask simple questions so that you will know how to troubleshoot a question you have asked nature but for which you can't get a clear answer. You'll know where your weaknesses in this area are and you'll be able to review the question to check for a problem.

As you develop internal order, your intuition will become clearer and stronger. You will see that when you ask a simple yes/no question, you will intuitively sense the answer or begin to "hear" nature answer before testing. This is a normal development. I recommend that you continue with the kinesiology testing as a verification that your intuitive or "overheard" answer is correct.

It is also helpful, especially in the beginning, to literally verbalize your questions out loud and not just think them. When we say something aloud, we tend to articulate it better than when we just think it. And I will ask something out loud if I'm a little tired and I need some extra sensory input (sound) to help me keep my focus.

FINAL COMMENTS ON KINESIOLOGY

Kinesiology is like any tool. The more you practice, the better you become at using it. You need a sense of confidence about using this tool, especially when you get some very strange answers to what you thought were pretty straight questions. It helps you get over the initial "this-is-weird-and-the-damned-testing-isn't-working" stage if you have some confidence in your ability to feel clear positive and negative responses. The only way I know to get over this hump is to practice testing. It is impossible to mentally reason yourself over the hump. Through practice you will develop clarity in your testing, you'll learn your personal pitfalls and you will fine-tune your technique.

In teaching kinesiology, I have found that something interesting happens to some people when they are learning it. Every block, doubt, question, concern and personal challenge they have, when faced head-on with something perceived as unconventional, comes right to the surface. It is as if the physical tool of kinesiology itself serves to bring to the surface all those hurdles. So they learn kinesiology right away and are using it well. Then, all of a sudden it is not working for them. When they tell me about it, I realize that the thing they do differently now that they didn't do at first is double-checking their answers—and rechecking, and rechecking, and doing it again, and again. . . . Each time the answers vary or the fingers get mushy and they get definite maybe's.

Well, again the issue is not the kinesiology. The issue is really why they are suddenly doing all this rechecking business. What has surfaced for them are questions around trust in their own ability, belief that such unconventional things really do happen and are happening to them. They have a sudden lack of self-confidence.

Again, the only way I know to get over this hurdle is to defy it—keep testing. Keep doing the co-creative processes. They all require testing and you will be able to observe the positive results. The successful results, in turn, give you

186

confidence about your testing ability. The other alternative is to succumb and stop developing kinesiology. But that doesn't really accomplish anything. So in cases like this, I suggest the person keep testing, *stop double-checking* and take the plunge to go with the first test result. Eventually, what action is taken based on the first test result will verify the accuracy of the test. As I've said, from this, your confidence builds. I firmly believe that only clear personal experience and evidence can get us through these kinds of blocks and hurdles—and that means just continuing to go on.

As I have worked through the years to refine my ability to use kinesiology, nature has provided many occasions when I have had to follow through on answers that made no sense at all to me. Doing this and looking at the results with a critical eye is the only way I know to learn about ourselves as kinesiology testers and to discover the different nuances and uses of kinesiology itself.

One last piece of information: Give yourself about a year to develop a strong confidence with kinesiology. Now, you'll be able to use it right away. This just takes sticking with your initial efforts until you get those first feelings of positive strength and negative weakness in the circuit fingers. But I have found from my experience and from watching others that it takes about a year of experimentation to fully learn the art of asking accurate yes/no questions and to overcome the hurdles. As one woman said, "You stick with this stuff a year, and boy, what a great thing you end up with!"

About Perelandra
and the Author

Perelandra is both home for my partner Clarence and me, and a nature research center. It now consists of forty-five acres of open fields and woods in the foothills of the Blue Ridge Mountains in Virginia. The nature research and development has been going on since 1976, when I dedicated myself to learning about nature in new ways from nature itself. I began working with nature intelligences in a coordinated and educational effort that has resulted in understanding and demonstrating a new approach to agriculture and ecological balance.

The primary focus of my work has been the 100-foot-diameter circular garden where I get from nature the information I need to create an all-inclusive garden environment based on the principles of balance. For example, we do not attempt to repel insects. Instead, we focus on creating a balanced environment that calls to it and fully supports a complete and appropriate population of insects. In turn, the insects relate to the garden's plant life in a light and nondestructive manner.

From this work has developed a new method of gardening that I call "co-creative gardening." Briefly, this is a method of gardening in partnership with the nature intelligences that emphasizes balance and teamwork. The balance is a result of concentrating on the laws of nature and form. The teamwork is established between the individual and the intelligent levels inherent in nature. Both of these point out the differences between co-creative agriculture, and traditional organic gardening and agricultural methods. (Information about this work is described in three books: *Behaving as if the God in All Life Mattered; Perelandra Garden Workbook: A Complete Guide to Gardening with Nature Intelligences;* and *Perelandra Garden Workbook II: Co-Creative Energy Processes for Gardening, Agriculture and Life.*)

The foundation of the work going on at Perelandra, as I have indicated, comes from nature intelligence. My work with flower essences and a number of physical health and balancing processes and programs has also been developed from this foundation.

As a result of the research with nature at Perelandra, a new science has developed called "co-creative science." Traditional science is man's study of reality and how it works. Co-creative science is the study of reality and how it works from nature's perspective and by man and nature working together in a peer, i/e (involution/evolution) balanced partnership.

My education has been only a part of what has gone on here. The fact that Perelandra is a research center and the garden its laboratory has given nature intelligence a place in which to work out the laws of nature—balance—in new ways that better address the environmental and health issues we presently face. Much of our published material is a result of this particular area of focus.

The term "research center" has caused many to think that we are a community and open to the public. We are not. We are a private research center and we have no plans to expand to a traditional community.

We feel it is important to maintain an environment that will facilitate and enhance the research: calm and quiet. The best way to accommodate the research as well as the many requests to visit Perelandra is to have several annual open houses during the summer and early fall. Aside from these open houses, Perelandra is closed to the public. We cannot accommodate unannounced or unscheduled visits. We appreciate your understanding in this and hope that the open houses address your need to visit and experience Perelandra.

We have had to consider how to maintain the proper research environment while we get information to others so that they may begin implementing it in their lives. It is a tricky balance. This is where our catalog and web site come in. There is much going on here and we feel our most efficient and effective means for sharing the Perelandra information is through the catalog and the web site. If you would like our catalog (there is no charge for it), here's how to contact us:

24-Hour Ordering Phone Numbers (answering machine)
U.S. and Canada: 1-800-960-8806
Overseas and Mexico: 1-540-937-2153
24-Hour Fax Line: 1-540-937-3360
Our address: P.O. Box 3603, Warrenton, VA 20188
And if you are a net surfer, you can get our entire current catalog plus other information: http://www.perelandra-ltd.com

We have a terrific staff who will respond to your request right away. We look forward to this vital outreach with you and hope there is something we offer that helps you in your personal understanding and relationship with nature.

BIBLIOGRAPHY

Books by Machaelle Small Wright
All books published by Perelandra, Ltd.

Behaving as if the God in All Life Mattered
(revised and updated edition)
*Perelandra Garden Workbook: A Complete Guide
to Gardening with Nature Intelligences*
(second edition)
*Perelandra Garden Workbook II: Co-Creative
Energy Processes for Gardening, Agriculture
and Life*
*Flower Essences: Reordering Our Understanding
and Approach to Illness and Health*
*MAP: The Co-Creative White Brotherhood
Medical Assistance Program*
(second edition)
Dancing in the Shadows of the Moon
Perelandra Microbial Balancing Program Manual